# ARTHRITIS

The Rowland Remedy

To
Beulah
Mark James
Olive and Pop

# ARTHRITIS

## The Rowland Remedy

John Rowland

JAVELIN BOOKS
POOLE · DORSET

First published in the UK 1985 by Javelin Books,
Link House, West Street, Poole, Dorset, BH15 1LL

Distributed in the United States by
Sterling Publishing Co., Inc.,
2 Park Avenue, New York, NY 10016

**British Library Cataloguing in Publication Data**

Rowland, John
 Arthritis : the Rowland remedy.
 1. Rheumatism—Treatment    2. Arthritis—
Treatment    3. Herbs—Therapeutic use
 I. Title
 616.7'2061            RC927

ISBN 0 7137 1609 6

Typeset by Cheney & Sons Ltd., Banbury, Oxon. England.

Printed in Great Britain by Guernsey Press

# Contents

# Acknowledgements

I would like to thank my colleagues, family and friends for their help in compiling this book, in particular Angus Thomas, BSC, CChem, FRSC, Christopher Thompson MIBiol, GRIB, AIB, ASAB, Valerie Anwyl and Alice and the late Harry Pollard.

# Addresses

General Council and Register of Consultant Herbalists, Villa Merlyn, 18 Elgin Road, Talbot Wood, Bournemouth BH4 9NL

National Institute of Medical Herbalists, School of Herbal Medicine, 148, Forest Road, Tunbridge Wells, Kent

Letters to the author will be most welcome and should be addressed to: The Naturopathic Private Clinic, 76 Victoria Road East. Cleveleys, Lancashire FY5 5HH    (0253 853482)

# Foreword

My acceptance to write the Foreword for this book was based on my progression from patient to a firm believer in 'alternative medicine' as practised by J.C. Rowland. It has also provided me with an opportunity to emphasise the importance of this book.

Initially, the reader's response may be a natural scepticism – 'Can it possibly work' – arising from years of affliction and doubt about ever finding the sort of relief offered in the book.

It is important therefore, at the outset, to outline my personal experience. For 30 years, I had learned to live with lumbago; it was part of my life as was the phrase 'Go to bed and see me in a week's time'. It was natural that I should be sceptical when I was introduced to John Rowland and was told after the examination that the condition could be relieved and would not re-occur. That was 8 years ago. There has been no re-occurrence.

What is equally important is that, during the course of the treatment (detailed in his book) John explained its basic principles. This aroused my curiosity and, during my continued association with him, I undertook a study of nutrition and dietetics – the requirements necessary to maintain the body in good health.

I now understand and confirm the principles used in this book and strongly recommend that the treatment programme should be considered seriously by the many people who are afflicted by arthritis in its various forms. It is important to remember that one cannot expect a disease which has taken many years to develop to be alleviated in days and therefore a patient, consistent application of the treatment is essential for a successful outcome.

Finally, a valuable benefit arises: in learning how to treat your affliction, you are also learning how to improve the state of your body generally so that it can maintain itself in a better, healthier condition.

*A.A.M. Thomas* FRSC

# Preface

People who visit herbalists tend to have chronic conditions which have failed to respond to conventional medicine as prescribed by their doctor, and it is often in desperation that they turn to someone like me. They are sometimes so disillusioned that they have very little confidence left in their ability to cope with life and the first thing I have to do is restore their confidence, both in themselves and in what they can expect from herbal treatment.

It usually surprises people, but certainly reassures them, to know that the training of herbalists today is rigorously controlled. In the UK, it is undertaken by the Faculty of Herbal Medicine and by the National Institute of Medical Herbalists, each body providing academic training leading to diploma qualifications. At the end of the course, there is a period of practical instruction from experienced medical herbalists. Both organisations are flourishing and ensure by their efforts that the high esteem in which British herbalism is held throughout the world is continued.

It should be pointed out that it is still not a legal requirement in the UK to be qualified before one may practise herbal medicine, although moves are being made in this direction. Because of this, I strongly advise any client seeking help to ask whether or not the practitioner they have in mind is qualified. The letters to look out for are MRH, which signifies that the holder is a registered medical herbalist who has undergone training with the Faculty of Herbal Medicine: this is the training section of the General Council and Register of Consultant Herbalists (address on

p. 6). The letters MNIMH signify that the practitioner has undergone training with the National Institute of Medical Herbalists and has become a member of that body (address on p. 6). Both organisations have graduates working in Canada, Australia and New Zealand.

In the UK, the growth of herbal medicine was given a boost by the introduction of the Medicine Act (1968). The previous Act had been lax enough to allow the release onto the market of drugs such as thalidomide, and so the new Act was passed. It gave the opportunity for the British Herbal Medicine Association, whose members include such well-known people as Hugh Mitchell, Fletcher Hyde, David and Tony Hampson and Marjorie and Kenneth Robinson, to have a clause included that ensured that medical herbalists had the freedom they required to develop their profession.

Since the new Medicine Act, the same stringent controls that are placed on the pharmaceutical industry are placed also on herbal preparations. The rigid quality control demanded by the Department of Health and Social Security (DHSS) or the Ministry of Agriculture, Fisheries and Food (MAFF) in the UK and the Food and Drug Administration (FDA) in the USA has undoubtedly improved the standard of preparations on the market, though the controls are not without their drawbacks for herbalists: the main problem is that most herbal knowledge is accumulated by observation rather than by clinical trials and, in order to satisfy the regulations covering the marketing of herbal preparations, one has to show scientifically how they work on the body's metabolism.

The fact that herbal medicine is based on knowledge accumulated over thousands of years is something I touch on when reassuring prospective clients about the respectability of the profession. Even today, much information is passed on from one individual to another and I, for example, have the privilege of having known some of the herbalists of an earlier generation who were responsible for keeping herbalism alive in Britain during a difficult period. C. Abbott, F. Power, J. Napier, E. Hackett and my good friend and colleague Lawrence Brimelow are some of them.

In an initial interview with my client, I have also to point out the limitations of herbalism. If I were involved in a car crash and required surgery of some kind then I would go to a surgeon for treatment; if I had any condition that would best be treated by the use of antibiotics then I would, and do, consult my local general practitioner. If, however, a condition is one of toxaemia or, like that of arthritis, psoriasis, hypertension, colitis or asthma, one of degeneration, then it is almost always worthwhile trying an holistic approach – herbal medicine integrated into a total health programme similar to the one explained in this book.

It may also be useful to continue some drugs prescribed by a doctor, as in an holistic approach it is not the means, but the end, which counts, and that end is eventual restored good health. The Chinese attitude to medicine is such that the patient can receive either herbal or orthodox medicine or, if appropriate, both. Nobody gets upset because of professional pride; each profession is respected for the contribution it is making to the individual's total health programme.

I look forward to the day when, in the West, professional prejudice is put aside for the benefit of the individual and hope that the information given in this book is a start in the right direction.

Certainly the information can be used in a number of ways. The holistic self-care programme which is described is designed specifically for the treatment of arthritis and can be followed at home, preferably in consultation with a family doctor. As an integral part of the treatment plan, detailed advice is given on how to eat sensibly (the Rowland Remedy Food Guide) and this can be used as a basis for healthy living generally. The final part of the book is a straightforward reference section, dealing with herbs, vitamins, minerals and trace elements and various important foodstuffs, and gives details of their sources, composition and health-giving properties. Taken as a whole, the book will give the reader an insight into the use of herbalism as part of an holistic form of treatment and also into the influence herbalism is having on modern medicine and society in general.

*John Rowland*
*Cleveleys,* 1985

# Part 1
# Introduction to the Alternative Approach

# 1 Herbal Medicine Today

The theory and principles that I put forward in this book are not new. Plant medicine in the cultures of ancient China and Egypt was one of the major sciences and, as a Hindu friend, Anil Hindocha, recently pointed out to me, the ancient Hindu medicine which was practised well before 1,000 BC was of the opinion that arthritis was a condition which was caused by a surplus of bile, phlegm, blood, fat or air. Treatment of the condition was to help the body establish good health by removing these excesses or toxins: to do this, herbal blood-purifying agents were used and perspiration was stimulated; in addition they used massage and a system of purging in an effort to break down the deposits of metabolic waste that had accumulated in the joints or muscles, or had built up into renal calculi (kidney stones).

Now, thousands of years later, I am presenting you with the same principles of detoxification in an effort to create a situation in which the body can heal itself. Our advantage over the Ancients is that we have the accumulated knowledge, ancient and modern, Eastern and Western, on which to base our treatment programmes.

As recently as the beginning of this century, almost all the medicines prescribed by doctors had their origins in the plant kingdom, many being dispensed in the form of extracts, or pills, or infusions, as we suggest in this book. Herbal medicine was trusted because it had evolved over thousands of years of trial and error.

When the pharmaceutical industry discovered its ability

14

to synthesise drugs from plant sources and mineral elements, herbal medicine lost favour because it was slower in action than the new, convenient and immediate preparations. The effect of the new drugs, even if dubious in relevance to the ailment, was to satisfy both doctor and patient, in the short term at least, as something was being achieved immediately.

The position of herbal medicine was further weakened by the discovery of antibiotics, probably the greatest gift to mankind this century, responsible for alleviating more suffering, and saving more life, than any other form of medicine. (It is of interest to note, however, that, if the massive need for penicillin had not arisen during World War 2, it had already been planned to extract and market the antibiotic properties of garlic on a commercial scale.) You need only stand in the outpatients' department of any hospital for a few minutes to be convinced of the need for the drugs and surgery of allopathic medicine, as orthodox Western medicine is termed, and yet there is a movement throughout the world rejecting many of these drugs in favour of a revival of interest in plant medicine. There is a desire for mild, natural cures which can be used in conjunction with an holistic approach to self-care.

I think this about-turn on the part of the public all over the world is the result of two basic factors. The first is that people are in general better educated than formerly and feel confident of their ability to take responsibility for their own health as far as is possible; the second is that the side effects of many drugs used in allopathic medicine are, or can be, much worse than the original condition for which they have been prescribed. These drugs have evolved in part because of a natural desire on the part of the public for a miracle pill in times of illness, with the medical profession believing, and allowing the public to believe, that such a thing is possible. The pharmaceutical industry seems to have been able to convince everybody, mainly by glossy advertising, that miracles can indeed be worked.

The public, however, has slowly come to realise that the only miracle that exists is the human body, and that it is the body's own defences that we should be helping wherever possible. The search for mild, effective medicine which has minimal side effects, is non-habit forming and which can be used in a self-care system is the dominant cause of a world wide resurgence of interest in herbs, vitamins, minerals and alternative therapies, a movement now so great that throughout the world it is being referred to as the 'green wave'.

Herbal medicines are natural substances derived from plants, whereas many allopathic drugs are synthetic chemicals. This is not the case with all of them, however, and many well-known orthodox medicines which have stood the test of time are derived from the plant kingdom. Countless people throughout the world owe their lives to an ornamental flower called foxglove (*Digitalis purpurea*), which doctors prescribe to correct irregular heart beats, strengthen the heart muscle contractions and prevent congestive heart failure. It acts by maintaining a healthy balance between the sodium and potassium in the heart cells.

A major success story of hospitals specialising in the treatment of cancer has been the breakthrough in the management of leukaemia and Hodgkin's lymphoma by the use of alkaloids. Alkaloids are nitrogenous substances occurring naturally in plants. They possess marked physiological properties and are often medicinally valuable. Some plants contain a very large number of alkaloids, and two of the sixty alkaloids present in the Madagascar periwinkle are being extracted: leukocristine which is active against leukaemia, and vincaleukablastine which is active against Hodgkin's lymphoma. They act by interfering with the assembly of tubulin, a protein which is essential to the structure and form of the cell, and so they slow down the rate of division of the cancer cell.

The fact that plant derivatives are so successfully used in some instances in orthodox medicine raises the question of why herbal medicine should so casually be dismissed out of hand by many practitioners of this allopathic medicine! It often comes as a surprise to people that the original source of aspirin was the willow bark which contains salicylic acid, its synthetic form being acetyl salicyclic acid. I use willow bark and meadowsweet tablets to help alleviate pain in the treatment of arthritis.

On the subject of pain, it is interesting to know that the herb curare, which the South American Indians use as poison in their blowpipes, has its use in most hospitals today; it contains an agent called tubocurarine which surgeons use to relax the muscles prior to an operation.

*Rauwolfia serpentina* has long been used by herbalists to reduce blood pressure. The alkaloids which do the work have been isolated and are in use all over the world helping people to lower their blood pressure.

Two herbs in particular have had a dramatic effect on the state of the world today. The first of these is cinchona which is the source of quinine and associated agents used in the treatment of malaria. Without this drug, explorers and poineers would not have survived very long, and progress into uncharted wilds would have taken much longer to accomplish. Missionaries regarded cinchona as an indispensable agent in their medicine chest and it quickly became known as Jesuits' bark, a name which survives today.

The other herb that has had such a wide-reaching effect on the society we live in is the Mexican wild yam, from which we obtain an agent called diosgenin, a precursor for many of the steroid-based preparations available today, not least of which is the contraceptive pill with all its connotations of freedom for women.

Herbal medicines are natural substances derived from

17

plants which are often used by the plant for purposes such as defence against attack by insects or being eaten by other members of the animal kingdom. They are substances manufactured by the plant for that particular purpose and are therefore outside the main biochemic pathways of proteins, fats and carbohydrates. The current orthodox approach is to isolate these secondary plant products and try and define their specific action on the body, thence creating a new drug which is a purely chemical substance. The herbalist differs radically in his approach, using the whole herb, or whole herbal extracts, in the belief that the secondary plant products are better administered to the body in the balance put there by nature. This is termed as being in its synergistic form, which herbalists believe will give the body all the benefits of the whole range of substances to be found in each plant. There are fewer side effects from this method of use but most of the benefits, particularly when used in conjunction with an holistic treatment programme such as the one advocated in this book. The variety of substances contained in a herb balances what might be the harsh effect of a powerful individual chemical. The plant *Ephedra* is used, for example, to treat asthma: the chemical ephedrine, which is the ingredient active against asthma, has the side-effect of raising the blood pressure, but other constituents of the plant, included in herbal preparations, counter the effect of the ephedrine on the blood pressure. In the use of ephedrine in orthodox medicine, high blood pressure is risked and, if encountered, treated by yet another drug.

It is reasonable to suppose that secondary plant products will make valuable contributions to medicine in the future. There can be as many as a hundred secondary substances in any one plant and, given that there are over 350,000 known species of plant in the world, and so far we have only a cursory knowledge of about 10,000 of them, there is remarkable scope for research.

To help in this field, the World Health Organisation has established an Institute in Rome. Many universities and teaching hospitals around the world are helping them with research and herbalists are contributing information. This pool of knowledge must help to advance the cause of natural medicine greatly in the coming years.

# 2 The General Concept

In a nutshell, the general concept of holistic treatment is to create a condition, by means of diet, fasting , hydrotherapy, vitamin and mineral therapy, herbal medicine and usage of any other therapy that can make a contribution, whereby the body's own healing process can work. We are creating a programme of treatment that includes as many known agents and therapies that the body may require to heal itself. As Hippocrates recognised, all those years ago, 'the body is the prime physician'.

In this book, I am explaining the Rowland Remedy relevant to arthritis: it is a successful way of controlling this condition providing you have the necessary life force and determination to follow the programme through. It is one of forty different programmes, called the Rowland Remedies, which are an accumulation of clinical observations and handed-down knowledge from my predecessors at the naturopathic private clinic which I run.

The concept of the programme is simple: you first detoxify the body by eliminating from your diet as many of the foods as possible that may be causing your toxic condition and, at the same time, you set about clearing away what is already there. You fast every seventh day and have special baths twice a week in between the fast days, in addition to your normal baths. After the special baths, you use a blend of oils to massage into the spine and affected areas.

To ensure that you are following the programme properly, we insist on a stipulated breakfast and lunch, but the evening meal is left very much to your own discretion. You are, however, given a guide to what you may or may not eat at this meal. This is called the Rowland Remedy Food Guide and you will find it on p. 70. Having sorted out the diet and general eating habits, so that the body is not only detoxifying itself but also regenerating, we try to help it along by the use of health foods, vitamins and minerals and herbal medicine. These are listed fully in Part 3 of this book.

Having set about the detoxification and supplementation programmes, we then consider the various therapies which are available, to see which ones are likely to make a contribution to your self-care system. It may be allopathic drugs from your doctor, exercise, acupuncture, osteopathy, physiotherapy, your chiropractor or some form of electrical treatment. It does not matter which one or ones you choose, providing that each is making a positive contribution to the improvement of your condition. Including the therapy in your self-care system, think of it as a tool in the toolbox: use each one as it is relevant to your immediate need.

It should be mentioned that undertaking your self-care treatment does not mean that you are no longer your general practitioner's patient, but the fact that you are assuming more responsibility for your own good health should leave him more time to help you with counselling, and it is to be hoped that he will be interested in the progress you are making.


## DETOXIFICATION

One of the first things that one must learn when beginning a self-care system of treatment is the principle of elimination and what is meant by the detoxification process which is so basic to the success of the programme. Fundamental to this is the fact that the body has four means of elimination: by faeces via the large intestine; by passing urine via the kidneys; by perspiration via the skin, and by exhalation by means of the lungs.

When the body's four means of elimination are not working properly, toxaemia arises and this becomes the basis of most degenerative diseases. Simple forms of toxaemia are coped with by evacuation (by diarrhoea or vomiting) or by biliousness when the liver returns toxins to the intestine via the bile duct. A more insidious form of toxaemia is when the liver is unable to cope with the poison and allows it to enter the bloodstream. The kidneys will be brought into play to filter the poison but if they are overworked they will have to call on the lungs to help out. We are all familiar with the person who has been drinking heavily and whose breath still reeks of alcohol. This occurs when the kidneys cannot cope and the lungs are brought into play.

When neither the kidneys nor the lungs are able to deal with the problem, then the skin and pores are called on to help eliminate and, in bad cases of drunkenness, to use the same example, body odour as well as breath odour can all too easily be detected. At this point, the body is just about coping in eliminating the excesses, but to do this it has first to have stimulated the endocrine glands to release some of their hormones in order to reinforce the elimination process. If the body has to do this on a regular basis then an endocrine imbalance is often the outcome. In effect, the constant strain put upon the body in having to eliminate toxins results in the body becoming 'run down'.

This is the basis for most degenerative disease, because when the body's defences are down the virus or mycotoxin can get a hold. Sometimes nutrients are not available to the organs of the body so that more cells die than are created and so we get an aging or degeneration of that organ.

The first conditions to make themselves known are the minor ailments, the odd ache or pain and that feeling of being one degree under and not on peak form. After a period of time these minor ailments manifest themselves into various forms of arthritis, hypertension, various skin conditions such as psoriasis and eczema and various internal inflammations, such as bronchitis and colitis.

So what causes toxaemia? It depends on the particular susceptibility of the individual, but it could be alcohol, sugar, artificial food colourings, preservatives, drugs or one of many others. Apart from these, there are over 2,000 chemicals and additives that we may come into contact with in our daily lives without our knowledge – such things as polishes, paints and glues, detergents, inks and so on. Stress can be another cause of toxaemia, often the last straw for the body's defences. One person will be more at risk from one particular toxin than another, and it is for this reason that an individual self-care system makes such good sense in the treatment of degenerative diseases.

What then is the best way to help the body use its own natural detoxifying methods? How can we best aid the processes of elimination?

The first thing to do, to ease the process of excretion, is to ensure that there is plenty of dietary fibre in our meals. Diets with a high fibre content have received a lot of publicity recently (though it should be said that nature-cure enthusiasts were until recently lone voices advocating this form of treatment) and it is easy to find out which foods are good in this respect. Wholewheat bread, whole grains and legumes, and plenty of fruit and vegetables are the prime factors. The Rowland Remedy Food Guide ensures that the intake of dietary fibre is adequate. The importance of fibre in the diet is that it acts rather like blotting paper when passing through the alimentary canal, taking up a lot of the debris and waste products. There is also the added benefit that it normalises the peristaltic action of the alimentary canal so that constipation is avoided.

After ensuring that we have sufficient dietary fibre, then we must look at the intake of fluids to ensure that the kidneys are not being over- or underworked. Remember that the kidneys are the blood's filters and the second of our four means of elimination. It is vital that we achieve the right quantity and quality of fluids in our treatment programme. I recommend lemon juice and water, or cider vinegar and water, to start the day, also the grape juice and water 24-hour fast every seventh day. Remember that water is nature's solvent and so, in the main, drinks based on water should be taken: these could be herbal teas such as chamomile, peppermint, rosehip, nettle or comfrey – there are many to experiment with, such as parsley piert or dandelion which also makes a delicious coffee. I make this point about water-based drinks because I often find patients drinking juice-only when on the programme and, though juices are permitted, they should not be taken in excess.

The next area of elimination is the skin and its function of perspiration. It takes only a moment's thought to realise that the skin is the largest organ of the body. It has many physiological functions, but the one that we are most concerned with here is the ability to perspire and in so doing reduce the body's toxic build-up. This natural ability should be encouraged to the utmost and we achieve this in the programme by the use of hydrotherapy – the special baths.

These special baths should be taken at least twice a week. The sea salt which they contain combines many natural elements and has beneficial properties, not least of which are those of healing and antisepsis. The French are great supporters of thalassotherapy (the treatment of disease by sea bathing and sea air) and they have shown how many people who are suffering with varying diseases can be helped by effective use of the sea's natural powers. We are not all in a position to get to a warm coast at a moment's notice, but we can add sea salt to our bath water and bring some of the sea's beneficial powers to our homes.

More will be said about the ingredients of the special baths on p. 62, but the general principle is that they should stimulate free perspiration. It is advisable to take your bath late, just prior to going to bed, when, after applying the oils to the spine and affected areas, you should wrap yourself in a bath robe to both aid and absorb the perspiration. The next day you will be pleasantly surprised at the invigorating effect of the bath and be ready to tackle your condition again.

The fourth method by which the body may eliminate toxins is by exhalation. We are all familiar with the smell of garlic on the breath or the person suffering with halitosis due to a gastric complication. The breath odour is caused by the body using the lungs as one way of detoxifying itself. It is with this in mind that the deep breathing exercises are recommended, aerobics if agile enough – but only under supervision, plenty of walking, which is my favourite, and swimming if your condition allows.

You will now have a basic idea of how detoxification works and will have begun to understand the importance of aiding this process when on a total health programme. Not only do we gain the benefit of a better oxygen supply to the bloodstream, and thereby the cells, but we also rid the body of the toxic build-up of salts and calcium which is necessary before we can begin to make progress on the healing programme.

Remember that an holistic programme is based on three premises. The first is to provide the body with all the nutrients that it could possibly need to put itself into good health. The second is to detoxify, removing all the poisons and accumulated debris from the system. The third is to improve the circulation so that the above two processes can work fully, with the cells receiving the nutrients and the waste products being carried from the cells and eliminated.

To achieve this threefold aim, we make full use of herbal medicine, vitamin and mineral supplements, hydrotherapy, exercise, and any other useful therapies available, in an effort to create a condition in which the natural healing processes of the body can work to our best advantage.

25

# 3 About Arthritis

Arthritis today is a widely publicised disease, although, in one form or another, it has affected human beings throughout history. Indeed it is one of the oldest traceable diseases known to mankind and chronic spinal arthritis has been identified in the skeletons of the ape men of 2 million years ago.

It appears to have become more prevalent in the last few decades, mainly because of the increased scientific awareness of the nature of the disease and the vastly improved diagnostic techniques of modern medicine.

It was in the second century AD that Galen first grouped the rheumatic diseases together and called them arthritis but it was left to an English doctor, in the 1860s, a Doctor Garrod, to differentiate between the two basic conditions – rheumatoid and osteo-arthritis.

In this chapter, we will look at what is meant by arthritis, in both its forms. Due to its holistic nature, the treatment programme that will be explained in this book, is suitable for both forms of the condition and it is therefore from an academic point of view that they will be discussed here.

Firstly, let me make it clear that arthritis is not a contagious disease like influenza or measles. There is a popular theory that people may have inherited a predisposition towards the disease from their parents and that, during their lifetimes, this may be exacerbated by factors, (e.g. infection, stress, fatigue, poor life style, toxic conditions, diet, draughts, work conditions, injury). Any bacterial disease, even when cured, may predispose to arthritis in later life, as can any of the other nine factors mentioned. The order in which these factors are listed is not significant as too few studies have been carried out to determine their relative importance. However, it should be mentioned that, in any total health programme, such as the one which we will be discussing, all these points should be examined to see whether you can improve your circumstances, for example by changing your diet or by reducing the amount of stress in your life, and thus improve the chances of a successful cure that much better.

## FORMS OF ARTHRITIS

Arthritis exists in many forms which are known by various names.

### BURSITIS

This is often called 'tennis elbow' or 'housemaid's knee' and is probably one of the earliest signs of a tendency to arthritis. It is caused by an inflammation of the bursa, a small sac which contains fluid and is usually situated between a tendon and the bone over which the tendon rides. This often occurs at the elbow and knee joints; hence the names.

### REITER'S SYNDROME

This is linked with arthritis and is a combination of conjunctivitis and urethritis; it usually affects young males for an indeterminate period ranging from weeks to months. It is a very painful condition, characterised by inflammation of the urethra and the delicate membrane lining of the eyelids.

### FIBROSITIS

This is an inflammation and soreness found in the soft tissue of the body as opposed to the joints specifically. It is often referred to as rheumatism, a term which covers a whole range of localised conditions, often brought about by some trauma, such as injury or by pursuing a sport where there is a prolonged strain put on muscular tissue. It may also be referred to as backache or lumbago. It responds well to the sort of treatment discussed in this book; indeed it generally responds so quickly that it is rarely necessary to complete a full course of treatment. Adopting a healthy life style is a good basis to live by as, with any of the conditions that go by the name of rheumatism or fibrositis, there is always a predisposition towards arthritis.

## OSTEO-ARTHRITIS

This is the most common form of arthritis and is really a wear-and-tear condition brought about by excessive wear on one or more parts of the body, e.g. the finger joints or the weight-bearing joints such as the knees, hips and spine. The condition is slow to progress and very painful. Often the first signs are structural changes in the articular cartilage of the joints, which loses its smoothness so that the joint becomes stiff and sometimes immobile in consequence.

It is mainly a condition of middle age and is more prevalent in women than men but it can occur at any age, particularly in sportsmen and women or people who have suffered some trauma, such as a car accident. Weight is best kept to a minimum for obvious reasons; the less weight the joints have to carry the better.

There are many practitioners who think this condition should be called osteo-arthrosis because it is a wear-and-tear condition involving hardening of the joint as opposed to an inflammation (*itis* denotes inflammation) which is rarely present.

## RHEUMATOID ARTHRITIS

This is a chronic inflammatory and degenerative disease which affects various organs of the body, including the joints. Joints that are affected may be deformed and painful with marked limitation of movement'.

To understand the physiology of rheumatoid arthritis, one must first understand a little anatomy and then the chemical process of inflammation and degeneration which occurs when the body's auto-immune system is either not coping or malfunctioning.


## THE AUTO-IMMUNE SYSTEM

The human body has a very complex system of self-defence against infection and disease known as the *auto-immune system*. It is organised and served by various organs and cells of the blood.

Normally if an invading bacterium or virus, say salmonella or a 'flu virus, enters the body, it is detected by

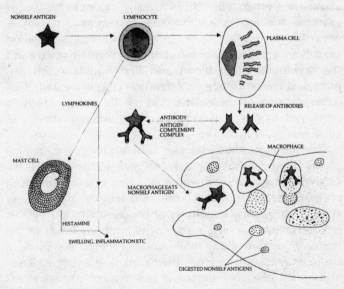

Figure 1. A schematic diagram of antigen-antibody reaction.

the first line of defence which is a type of white blood cell called a *lymphocyte*.

The lymphocyte's role is to distinguish anything it encounters in the blood or tissue as belonging to 'self' or 'non-self'. If it encounters 'self' then nothing occurs but when a foreign body or 'non-self' item ('non-self' antigen) is found, the body's immune system is triggered and a sequence of events is set in motion.

Initially, the lymphocytes that have encountered and recognised this non-self antigen are stimulated and start to produce a series of chemicals, *lymphokines*, which have several major effects. Initially, these lymphokines attract a different clan of white blood cells, called *macrophages*, whose job it is eventually to eat and digest non-self antigens by a process known as *phagocytosis*: this effectively negates any harmful properties of the non-self antigen.

The lymphocyte's lymphokines also have the job of stimulating other cells into producing more chemicals: for example, the mast cells will release histamine. This release of further chemicals causes a localised constriction of blood vessels around the site of infection, producing swelling and the accumulation of blood and body fluids – thus an increased concentration of defending cells is created. This often causes an immobilisation of the area which is perceived to the senses as swelling, inflammation and stiffness.

The stimulated lymphocytes now undergo a metamorphosis, changing into a much enlarged and aggressive cell known as a *plasma cell* whose function is to manufacture specific chemicals against the non-self antigens. These specific chemicals, known as *antibodies*, attack only this one particular non-self antigen: the antibody binds to the non-self antigen along with another blood chemical, a complement, and together they start destroying it. They also act as a beacon, signalling to the macrophages to eat and destroy it. In this way, the non-self antigen is neutralised and finally destroyed by these macrophages acting as vacuum cleaners and removing them from the body.

## THE JOINTS

A joint is the flexible junction of skeletal bone. The function of the joint is to allow a smooth and gliding movement of a limb. This is achieved by the encapsulation of two bone ends in a structure called the *synovium*. In effect, the ends of the bones are encased in a sealed lubricated environment; the lubricating fluid, called *synovial fluid*, contains glycoproteins, which are molecules made of sugar and protein, and certain blood cells. Also present within this capsule are cushions between the bone ends to stop them grinding together. These cushions are called cartilage.

In an arthritic joint, inflammation and degeneration of the bone ends is called *osteo-arthritis*, and inflammation and degeneration of the synovial membranes is *rheumatoid arthritis*.

## THE AUTO-IMMUNE SYSTEM AND THE JOINTS

In the person suffering from rheumatoid arthritis, an error has occurred in the first line of defence against the non-self antigens. Due to as yet unknown factors, the first line of defence in some persons has become confused and the normally helpful lymphocytes found within the synovial fluid perceive the bone ends or the synovial membranes as non-self antigens. Thus the body's defence system is put into action against these joint components which have been falsely identified as non-self antigens.

The lymphocytes produce their lymphokines which stimulate histamine release from the mast cells, thus causing swelling of the joints.

The lymphocytes metamorphose into plasma cells and

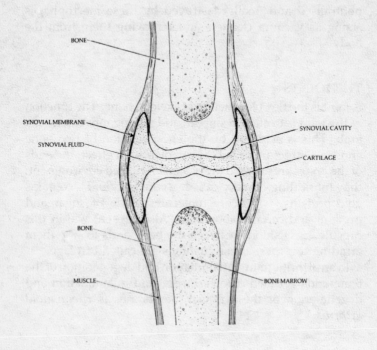

BONE

SYNOVIAL MEMBRANE

SYNOVIAL FLUID

BONE

MUSCLE

SYNOVIAL CAVITY

CARTILAGE

BONE MARROW

Figure 2. A typical synovial joint.

produce antibodies against the bone or synovial membranes. The attracted macrophages start to eat and digest the bones or synovial membranes, causing inflammation and degradation of tissue. The joint becomes swollen, stiff and painful to move, and eventually immobile. In severe cases, degeneration of the joint occurs.

This attack of the bone or synovial membranes causes the classic symptoms of arthritis, but because the human body contains systems for repair of damaged tissue, it starts trying to repair the very tissue the immune system is destroying. Thus an equilibrium between destruction and repair is struck and on the bias of the equilibrium depends the severity of the arthritic condition. This equilibrium may be tilted in either direction by environmental factors or by the general state of health of the individual.

The mistaken release of the lymphokines and agents of defence against the membranes and bone unfortunately may not be localised to a specific joint: it may spread throughout the body in varying degrees as the agents of defence leak from the joint into the bloodstream and find new joints and membranes: thus a person with an arthritic knee may suffer with a stiff neck or sore chest. This is known as the systemic effect of arthritis and is the reason why the pain appears to move around the body from muscle to muscle and joint to joint.

Where the joint has degenerated beyond the point at which one can reasonably expect the body's own repair mechanisms to work then surgery may be considered. Following the programme will certainly help, even if one has to recourse to surgery, as the total health programme will assist in the recovery period and subsequently in slowing down any further degeneration of the bone.

The most common replacement operation is the hip joint and its successs rate is extremely high. It results in tremendous relief for people with a disturbing degree of pain.

Modern pharmaceutical science has offered many 'cures' for arthritis, which in some cases have failed and in others have been very destructive of the general health of the patient. This is quite understandable considering that, in trying to suppress or remove the confused response, toxic drugs, by their very nature, also suppress the normal immune response.

There are, of couse, many rigorous safeguards throughout the world before any drug can be put on the market. Unfortunately, however, this has not stopped some slipping through the net in occasional cases, with disastrous consequences. The anti-arthritis drug Opren has recently been withdrawn after causing severe side effects, as have the painkillers Zomax and Osmin. There are a considerable number of other drugs that have been withdrawn, as well as many which have unpleasant if not dangerous side-effects. It is for this reason that more and more people are turning to alternative medicine for treatment.

In the next chapter, we will discuss our approach to the problem of remedying the confused body response and show how the use of herbs containing natural anti-histamines and anti-inflammatory and adrenal agents will help reduce pain and swelling while preserving the normal immune response to foreign invaders. Essentially we look at the body as a whole and use every means in our power to restore a healthy equilibrium in all the body's functions.

# Part 2
# The Alternative
# Approach

# 4 The Dietary Concept

In the creation of my treatment programme, I had several basic premises which I would like you to understand. Later in the book, I deal with individual foods, vitamins, minerals and herbs, but here I would like to outline the fundamental concept at the heart of the dietary part of your programme.

A good balance of amino acids, the body's basic building blocks, is essential; from this it will be able to synthesise its proteins. Secondly, a natural emulsifier is required to prevent the build-up of fats in the arteries. Thirdly, we should create as nearly as possible what I like to call a 'ninety-two element diet': a diet comprising all the elements of which the earth, of which you and I are a part, is composed. Fourthly, every seventh day we should undertake a 24-hour fast.

Combining the above four principles with our modern knowledge about the effects of individual foodstuffs and elements on particular functions of the body, we can come up with a practical general guide as a basis for our diet programme. This guide reduces to an eight-point plan and, if you keep this in mind, you will not go far wrong in selecting suitable foods for yourself. Until you are completely familiar with the composition of the foods you eat, however, it is difficult to be sure that your diet is perfect in all respects and it is for this reason that, on the programme, the breakfast and lunch menus are stipulated, leaving only the evening meal to your own discretion. You are asked only to follow the general guidelines and the eight-point plan which is as follows: high potassium content; low sodium content; low sugar content; low saturated fat content; high fibre content; high pantothenic acid (Vitamin B$_5$) content; rich sources of nutrients; known peculiarities of certain foods.

Very briefly, the reasons for these criteria are as follows. Potassium is essential to the body and one of the main agents we are striving to increase in our health programme. Often the body's potassium level is depleted, mainly by the excessive use of sodium, sugar and caffeine, by using diuretics too often, or by the factor so commonly underlying countless diseases – stress. People with arthritis, hypertension, leukaemia, heart disease, epilepsy and diabetes all have a depleted potassium level, often with a correspondingly high sodium level. Most of the body's potassium is found in the cells, with a small amount in the body fluids and bloodstream. It has many roles to play, of which an important one is to help maintain a normal heart rhythm; others are the maintenance of muscle tone and the formation of extra bone, although its precise role in this is not fully understood. Further information on potassium can be found on p.114.

At one time, there was a higher proportion of potassium than sodium in our diets and, indeed, the body adapted many of its own mechanisms to retain sodium: one of the functions of the kidneys is to ensure that the minerals are in the correct balance. However, there is such a high level of sodium in our present-day diets that our bodies are being overloaded with this mineral. In the Rowland Remedy Food Guide we try to redress the balance in our food intake to a level that the body can cope with: we do not try to ban it altogether. (See also p. 115 for further information on sodium.)

We try to keep our sugar intake low so that the body is encouraged to obtain part of its energy from naturally balanced carbohydrates – the complex carbohydrates, rather than the simple carbohydrate found in refined sugar.

The refining of carbohydrate has created virtual power packs of concentrated energy – in fact many products are sold on just this point – but it is really only when undertaking strenuous exercise that this sort of energy source is required. Most of us should strive to obtain our energy requirements from a mixture of complex carbohydrates, fats and protein, all of which are interchangeable as far as the body is conerned as an energy source. We should avoid as far as possible the simple carbohydrates, such as dextrose, fructose and sucrose. Carbohydrate is, of course, essential to the human brain, nerve and lung tissue, and is supplied to these areas in the form of glucose. The main problem associated with a high intake of sugars is that the excess is converted to fats (triglycerides) and stored in the body in the adipose tissue as fat. On this programme, any excess fat is bound to create a problem and overweight can lead to all sorts of complications in your condition.

We strive on the programme to lower the overall intake of fats and to guide you towards the use of less saturated fats. Fats are composed of two basic types of fatty acids: saturated (hard) and unsaturated (soft, oil-like). Natural fats are a mixture of saturated and unsaturated fatty acids. The unsaturated fatty acids are so named because of the incomplete portions of the molecule (double bonds) and may have between one and four double bonds per molecule. Those with one double bond are known as mono-unsaturated and those with two to four double bonds are known as poly-unsaturated; in this latter category are the essential fatty acids (linoleic, linolenic and archidonic acid) which are required for normal health but cannot be made in the body. Enough of these fatty acids should be present in the diet to provide approximately 2% of the energy intake. The greater the number of double bonds in the fat the more soft or oil-like is its consistency and, in order to incorporate these fats in foodstuffs to give a product which has an acceptable appearance and consistency, it is necessary for manufacturers to hydrogenate them, i.e., to saturate some or all of the double bonds to give a harder fat. The prime source of unsaturated fats is fish and vegetable oils, with the major exception of coconut oil, which is classed as saturated. We should be trying also to reduce our intake of artificially-created, hydrogenated, fats. This is very convenient for the food-producer who can thus virtually dictate the shelf-life of his product, but the end product is by no means ideal for us and should be avoided as much as possible.

The reasons for a high fibre intake have been discussed in the chapter on detoxification, but I would like to add here that evidence is accumulating all the time to support the advisability of adopting a diet rich in fibre such as bran. Oat bran, for example, contains an agent called $\beta$-glucan, which carries cholesterol to the colon, and serious medical conditions such as haemorrhoids, diverticulitis, varicose veins, colitis, cancer and atherosclerosis can all be attributed in some degree to a longterm lack of consumption of fibre.

Pantothenic acid (Vitamin $B_5$) is essential for the proper dispersal of fats, carbohydrates and proteins. It plays a major role in the creation of amino acids, sterols and steroid hormones and it is for this main reason that it is an important ingredient of our programme. There is further information on this substance on p.100.

In our treatment programme, it is essential that we provide the body with the raw materials from which it may select its own requirements and, for this reason, it makes sense to include in our diets foods which are rich sources of nutrients. Kelp, for example, contains many, many minerals and we would do well to study which foods are good sources of some of the more obscure minerals, such as manganese. The reference section of this book (pp.83-125) discusses which foods supply which vitamins and minerals.

In the Rowland Remedy Food Guide, we have taken into account clinical observations on patients suffering with arthritis and we have listened to the opinions of patients who have learned through trial and error which foods, food colourings and preservatives and methods of preparation have been counter-productive. The Food Guide reflects a balance of evidence for and against certain substances. Remember, however, that the essence of the self-care programme is that it is individually tailored and you will have to observe very carefully the effects of all foods and food substances on your own condition.

As it is important that you should fully understand the reasons behind the diet programme, let us now look in more detail at the fundamentals of the regime; the inclusion of amino acids, an emulsifier, the 'ninety-two element diet' and the fast.

Amino acids are, as already mentioned, the body's basic building blocks and they are obtained from our intake of protein. There are twenty-two of them, ten of which are essential to life. These are: arginine, histidine, isoleucine, leucine, lysine, methionine, phenylalanine, threonine, tryptophan and valine.

Unlike plants, which can manufacture their own proteins, we need to obtain proteins from food and it is essential that we have a regular intake of complete proteins from such things as lean meats, fish, eggs, fowl, milk, cheese, buttermilk, yogurts, soya beans, nuts, beans, peas, yeast and grains. As the egg has a near-perfect balance of amino acids, other sources of protein are compared with it as a reference standard. Unfortunately, the kidneys may have difficulty in coping with the high albumen content of eggs, so you should not have more than three eggs a week. Also there is the point that your amino acid intake is best obtained from a variety of sources so that thousands of different proteins can be manufactured by the body from the different amino acids broken down by the enzymes in the digestive process.

These amino acids are carried around the body by the

bloodstream and are selected by the cells for use in the production of new body tissue and replacement of such important substances as antibodies, hormones, enzymes and blood cells. It is easy to see that a long-term shortage of protein creates a condition in which degenerative disease can easily set in. (It should be mentioned in passing that a very high intake of protein over a long period can be injurious to health as damage in the form of nephritis can occur. Our need for protein varies very little whether we are at work or rest and any excess, over and above that needed for replacing the body tissue, puts a strain on the kidneys. In the stipulated diet, and following the eight-point plan for the selection of food, you should run no risk of overconsumption of protein.)

The second fundamental ingredient in our diet after amino acids is a natural emulsifier in the form of an element called lecithin. It is included as one of the regular ingredients of the breakfast in the treatment programme.

Most people will be aware of the danger of cholesterol deposits on the walls of the arteries. These deposits not only impede the flow of fresh, nutrient-rich blood to the cells but also become a danger to good health in themselves as the cause of heart disease. We must take steps in our diet not only to prevent the build-up of fat deposits, but also to clear away what is there at the present time.

Although cholesterol is always given a bad press, I should perhaps mention that it is constantly manufactured in the body by the liver in the right amounts to utilise Vitamin D and the hormones and bile salts it requires. It is rarely this type of cholesterol, however, that gives us problems with deposits on the artery walls. The troublesome sort comes from animal fats and processed foods containing hard or saturated fats and oils which have been hydrogenated. If the body finds no use for these globules of fat, they gather together in clusters on the artery walls and become the initial cause of conditions like high blood pressure,

41

hardened arteries, various heart diseases and strokes.

What is needed to break down these clusters is an emulsifier, a substance which acts as a sort of soap. Vegetable oils, such as sunflower and safflower, are bonded with lecithin, nature's strongest emulsifier, whose job it is to break down the globules of fat into small particles so that they are ready to be absorbed by the tissues when required.

As well as supplementing the diet with lecithin in granule form, it is wise to restrict the intake of fat to the polyunsaturated kind where lecithin is naturally present. It is interesting to note, as a bonus, that lecithin contains two important vitamins of the B complex, choline and inositol, essential to the brain, nerves, heart, lungs and in the production of certain hormones. It is also gaining a reputation as an agent that can prevent senile dementia.

The third premise on which our treatment programme is founded is that we should approach as nearly as possible a 'ninety-two element diet'. Trace elements are substances essential to plant or animal life but are present in only very small amounts. There are at least ninety-two of them and they make up the basic composition of the earth and everything in it. In that the same concentrations of salts and trace elements that make up our blood and tissues were found in the earliest seas – the primaeval soups – we can indeed be called the children of the earth. The nitrogen in the atmosphere that is 'fixed' by conversion in the soil to nitrates to feed plants is the same nitrogen that is part of the connective tissue that binds our bones together, just as the calcium in our bones is the same as the calcium that forms the rocks of our hills and mountains.

If we organise ourselves properly, then we should never be short of minerals as they are available in abundance. They are discussed in detail in the reference section on p.109, but it is worth mentioning here an obvious and balanced source of many nutrients. While we are still not sure what life is, we can at least see for ourselves the first act of growth of an embryo plant – the sprouting or germination of the seed. Although to sustain growth, it will need nutrients from water, soil and air, this initial surge of activity is supported entirely by the miniature chemical factory called the seed, in which all the natural elements are contained in the right proportions. As it is a source of balanced nutrients that we are trying to capture in our diet, it must make sense to include a high proportion of these basic forms of life; seeds, whole grains and legumes.

Fourthly, and finally as a general principle, a 24-hour fast is part of the treatment programme. The thinking behind this is that the body needs a period in which the elimination processes may be helped, and that the kidneys can have a chance to utilise the healing and diuretic properties of grape juice over that period. The Swiss have long regarded grape juice as a way of avoiding kidney stones, and the maintenance of healthy kidneys is one of our main aims on the programme.

The easiest way to achieve a 24-hour fast is to miss the evening meal of one day and the breakfast and midday meal of the next. The gap in eating is then spread over 2 days and no single day is spent without food.

# 5 An Holistic Approach

To remind you of the general concept of holistic treatment, we are looking to create a condition whereby the body can heal itself. In addition to the very important subject of diet, we can select from the variety of therapies which are available to aid blood circulation and the efficient function of heart and lungs. Some therapies, such as acupuncture, osteopathy, or chiropractic may also directly alleviate pain and they should be used where they can be helpful to our progamme. Before undertaking an holistic programme you should have a confirmed diagnosis of your condition from your doctor and his approval of the therapies you intend to use. You should review your self-care programme and take further medical advice if any sudden change occurs in your condition, particularly in the heart or lung function. In addition you should not continue with any aspect of your programme which you approach with a negative attitude so that you doubt its worth.

In the treatment programme, I stipulate the use of hydrotherapy, special baths and aromatherapy (the massage of oil into the skin) but other therapies available for consideration include deep breathing, exercise, homeopathy, acupuncture, osteopathy, chiropractic, physiotherapy or some form of electrical treatment. In addition, you may wish to use some allopathic drugs from your doctor.

Let us take a look in turn at each of these possibilities, starting with the ones I stipulate on the programme.

## HYDROTHERAPY

The idea behind the special baths is that they should stimulate free perspiration, thus aiding the process of elimination. In this arthritis programme, they are recommended twice weekly.

Have the bath water as hot as you can stand and add to it ½ lb (250 g) sea salt, ½ lb (250 g) Epsom salts and ½ oz (15 g) powdered ginger (ordinary culinary ginger). Keep the temperature of the bath water high by topping it up while you are soaking. Stay in the bath for at least 20 minutes.

When you get out of the bath, lightly dry yourself and, with the help of an assistant if necessary, apply Rowlo Oil to the whole of the spine and the affected areas (see the section below on aromatherapy). Then wrap yourself in a bath robe and retire to bed where you should perspire freely, aiding the elimination process.

As already mentioned, the properties of sea salt are many and varied. It is included in the special bath principally for its healing and antiseptic properties. 98% of known germs are unable to survive longer than 48 hours in sea water. The Epsom salts are included because of their healing and drawing properties when combined with sea salt and the ginger has the property of stimulating perspiration and toning the skin, which is the aim in the elimination part of the programme.

It is advised that you have the bath water as hot as you can stand. Apart from the fact that any source of heat often alleviates arthritic pain, the heat will aid the elimination process, as will the emergence into a steamy atmosphere. It also helps in the softening of any intramuscular salt deposits which may be causing lesions. It is suggested that the special bath is taken twice weekly as a minimum. It may be taken more often if desired, particularly if you have pain and find that the bath alleviates this for you. Do not, however, take a special bath on the fast days: the drawing and cleansing effect of the bath will also lower your blood sugar level and you may feel a little drained for a short period afterwards, although delighted with the results the following day when you will feel lighter and more mobile. The combination of the fast and the bath together can lower the blood sugar level too much and result in your becoming dizzy and weak.

There is an exercise which can be undertaken in a special bath which helps to relax the spinous process. It relaxes the back muscles from top to bottom, allowing tension to be released on the spine. Small adjustments can then take place naturally that would not otherwise have been possible. Add the sea salt, Epsom salts and ginger to 3–4 in (8–10 cm) of very hot bath water. Now lie flat on the bottom of the bath with your hands by your sides and your knees bent so the soles of your feet are flat on the bottom of the bath. Now relax and work the head from side to side until there is a release in tension, which you will hear. Now bring your knees towards the chin and hold for 30 seconds. After doing this, sit up in the bath, raise the water level and relax for 20 minutes. Finish off your bath by applying oil to the spine and affected areas. A useful tip is to put a little cotton wool with a spot of olive oil in the ears before taking the bath. This stops any of the bath additives, such as ginger, getting in the ears.

## AROMATHERAPY

The massage of Rowlo Oil into the spine and affected areas strictly comes under the heading of a form of treatment called *aromatherapy* – the massage into the skin of a blend of essential oils. It is based on the knowledge that individual essential oils have particular effects on particular functions of the body. Aromatherapy is a fascinating subject and one that it is particularly pleasant to experiment with.

I give on p. 77 the ingredients of Rowlo Oil. My main

concern in formulating this oil was to include as many of the healing properties of different oils as one possibly could into one oil. The formula is based on one that was given to me by an Indian herbalist; it is beneficial without being as greasy as most other oil combinations.

You do not have to restrict the use of this therapy to just after your special baths. You may practise it at any time.

If you wish to experiment further, there are many books available on this subject which describe in detail massage techniques and also the properties of particular oils.


## THE AIR YOU BREATHE

Daily deep breathing exercises will ensure that your lungs are used to the full every day. You should take any opportunity that presents itself during the day to breathe good fresh air and expand the lungs to the full to help your tissues get their much needed oxygen.

Let us now pay some attention to the air we are breathing in, as this is so important to good health and indeed to life itself.

You have no doubt been in rooms where the air feels stifling. This may not in fact be due to poor ventilation, but rather to the dearth of negative ions in the air.

All air contains electrically-charged particles, positive and negative ions, and it is the negative ions in the air that are important to good health. What we perceive as stuffiness is a dearth of negative ions in the air, leading to a heavy feeling which drains the energy. Negative ions are produced in nature by the ultra-violet rays of the sun, reactions in soil, in water when droplets split, and lightning. The air is so bracing in the countryside and at the sea because of an abundance of negative ions.

If you do not live in the country or at the sea, or even if you do and you have central heating, it is quite likely that the air you breathe has a depleted level of negative ions.

There is, perhaps surprisingly, something you can do about this. There are on the market today many varieties of a gadget called an ioniser. It can be found in all shapes and sizes and is available in models suitable for home, office and cars. It plugs into a socket and uses very little electricity indeed, about 2% of that used by a single light bulb. Models vary in price but are available from as little as the cost of a good pair of shoes.

## EXERCISE AND RELAXATION

As well as the exercise for relaxing the spine which we saw under the heading of hydrotherapy, and the deep breathing exercises described above, you may like to consider walking and swimming, or more formal types of exercise such as yoga or aerobics. If you wish to try either of the latter, do so only under the guidance of an expert teacher and make sure that he knows the details of your condition. It is also worth mentioning to your doctor that you wish to take up some form of exercise.

For the more incapacitated who are following the programme, isometric exercise may be helpful. There have been many books written about these various systems of exercise, and because of this I will not go into detail about any of them. The general rule, however, is that where you feel that they are doing you good and that you are enjoying them, then continue. If you are in pain with them then stop them and try an easier form of exercise until such time as you have improved sufficiently to restart the ones of your choice.

Do not, under any circumstances, stretch or overwork any muscle or joint in the belief that the more pain that you have the more it is beneficial to the healing process. This is not the case. It is much more important to adopt a gentler approach on a regular basis to improve your circulation and improve your mobility.

# HOMEOPATHY

Dr Hahnemann in the nineteenth century developed his theory of homeopathy into what has become today a very popular form of medicine. The British Royal Family have been ardent supporters of it for four generations.

The principle is that the body, when experiencing an illness, produces symptoms, e.g. headaches, dizzy spells, a rise in temperature, skin rashes, etc. and, Hahnemann maintained, these symptoms are the manifestation of the body striving to put itself right; therefore, he suggested, a treatment should make the symptoms worse for a short period before there is an improvement in the general condition. The treatment should be a homeopathic remedy which has previously produced similar symptoms when tried out on a healthy individual.

As with herbalism, the total approach will be used by the practitioner who will take into account the patient's spiritual, mental, emotional and physical needs before assessing which remedy to prescribe. He will enquire about work and home life, eating and sleeping habits, allergies and medical history.

The method of preparing homeopathic remedies is to take the 'mother tincture' and potentise the solution. Take one drop of the mother tincture and add to it nine drops of solution; this is shown as $1\times$. One drop of the $1\times$ solution is then added to nine drops of the solution and this is shown as $2\times$. One drop of $2\times$ is then added to nine drops of the solution and this is shown as $3\times$, and so on until you reach the titration required. Thus the amount of original tincture is very small by the time it gets to the patient.

Nobody is sure how this form of treatment works, but it certainly does. When a cholera epidemic spread through Europe in the nineteenth century, patients treated by homeopathic remedies had a much higher survival rate than those treated allopathically.

## ACUPUNCTURE

Acupuncture has been practised for at least 5,000 years and has currently become fashionable throughout the world, the present revival being stimulated by Mao Tse Tung's 'barefoot doctors' in the 1950s.

The principle of acupuncture is to ensure that the life force, which flows through the body along channels called meridians, is maintained at its peak. This is achieved by inserting needles into various points along these channels to try to balance the flow of energy (referred to as 'chi') and thereby attack the cause of disease.

More recently it has been discovered that needles stimulate the brain into releasing substances called endorphins which are naturally produced painkillers with a marked similarity to morphine. Now that a scientific basis has been established for this form of treatment, many hospitals are now setting up pain clinics and are using acupuncture in them.

## OSTEOPATHY

Osteopathy is based on the theory that mechanical faults in the structure of the body are responsible for many illnesses.

The object of the treatment is to restore movement in the spine or joint so as to free any trapped nerves and restore full blood supply to the area, thus allowing the body's own healing process to act on the disease.

The originator of the theory of osteopathy was Andrew Still, who had the unusual distinction of being both a doctor and an engineer. This led him to the conclusion that the relationship between structure and function is paramount to good health. He began to treat patients by manipulation towards the end of the nineteenth century and opened his first training school in 1892 at Kirkville, Missouri. The method quickly spread round the world with the first training school in the UK being established in 1914, just before the war. The practitioner will attempt to restore normal movement by manipulation of the joint and leverage in such a manner as to allow both the muscles and ligaments to adjust as well as the joint: a thrust action is often used, particularly in the lumbar roll, a movement often used by osteopaths in the treatment of lower back disorders.

## CHIROPRACTIC

Chiropractors concentrate on the spine in their treatments in much the same way as the osteopath does, by manipulating the muscles and joints to establish equilibrium by improving the circulation and freeing the nervous system.

They tend to use more aids, such as X-rays, than the osteopath and they use a manipulative technique of short lever, quick thrust as opposed to the long lever and rotating-type thrust of the osteopath.

The success of chiropractic has been suggested by popular support mainly in the USA but now also in Europe, New Zealand and Canada. There are over 25,000 practitioners in the USA and they have over 40 million clients per year which is sure testimony to the success of their treatments.

In undertaking chiropractic therapy, as with acupuncture and osteotherapy, you would benefit more from a course of, say, ten sessions than by having sporadic bursts of treatment.

## PHYSIOTHERAPY

Your doctor may well refer you to a consultant who will be able to arrange physiotherapy for you. Massage, manipulation, and applied local heat, often by electrical methods, are his staple tools. He will also recommend a series of home exercises to do between treatments. The physiotherapy departments of hospitals are doing magnificent work in this area but are all too often overworked, and you may be better finding a private practitioner in this field.

The therapies described above are the the types of treatment that I feel you will find most useful to include in your treatment programme. You may find that one therapy helps you better than others, in which case this is the one for you. It does not mean that the others are no good, just that they do not help your particular case.


## ALLOPATHIC MEDICINE

Orthodox medicine in the West is referred to as allopathic, a word which derives from the Greek words *allos* 'other' and *pathos* 'suffering'. It is the method of treating disease by the use of agents which produce effects different from the diesase being treated. It thus takes the opposite standpoint from homeopathy.

The basic premise on which the doctor will be working is to reduce the pain and enable the patient to lead as normal a life as possible. He will be employing the supportive role of the physiotherapist and he will be prescribing analgesic and anti-inflammatory drugs. This is, of course, a very different approach from the one I am putting forward in this book, but it can work in parallel with a self-care treatment programme with considerable success.

# 6 The Living Proof

You must believe and persevere in your own management towards the relief of arthritis. There will be stages in the programme which follows when it is difficult to believe that you are making any progress, and it is for this reason that I now include comments from patients of mine which demonstrate typical feelings at various stages of the treatment and, happily, typical relief at the eventual cure. The letters are representative of the many hundreds of people who have attended my clinic and have derived benefit from the system of medicine called the Rowland Remedies which has evolved over the years into one of total health and self-care, relevant, with variations, to the treatment of many ailments, including psoriasis and hypertension. To use a system of this nature requires effort, but the reward of good health it brings is priceless.

Virtually all the people that come to me have tried treatment by orthodox medicine and, although the treatment may have failed, there is an advantage in that, in every case, records exist to show that the condition has a confirmed diagnosis. The type of treatment used prior to the consultation with me is also on record and it is very helpful for me to have a positive relationship with the patient's medical adviser, though this, unfortunately, does not always develop.

Some points you should note when reading the letters are the different times it takes to see results; the amount of tablets and liquid medicine which is taken; the fact that all the ingredients can be purchased from your health food store or products agent; and the importance of good nutrition to the success of the programme. Details of stockists can be obtained from the Naturopathic Private Clinic (see *Addresses*, p. 6).

At the Naturopathic Private Clinic, I have clients from as far afield as the USA, South Africa, Nigeria and Saudi Arabia, which is amazing when you consider that no advertising is undertaken, all recommendations being by word of mouth.

Following a discussion with one of my clients, Mrs H. decided that a natural treatment was also for her. She consulted her doctor, who had no objections and, indeed, co-operated by monitoring her progress on the programme. He gradually reduced her treatment for arthritis and hypertension as her condition improved. One further point to note here is that colitis is often present as a further complication in the arthritic with high blood pressure; all the symptoms of this quickly disappeared in this case.

I had suffered with arthritic knees for over twenty years, during which time my doctors gave me various tablets which helped ease the pain. Then unfortunately I developed colitis and could not take any pills as these aggravated this condition. I also started to suffer from high blood pressure and had to start taking tablets which my doctor said I would have to take for the rest of my life.

The arthritis became much worse: going upstairs, walking up even slightly hilly streets, and kneeling became a bit of a nightmare, and I grew tired and depressed with the effort. I also got increasing pain in my shoulders, arms and top of my spine which kept me awake most nights. At this stage a friend of mine recommended Mr Rowland and he put me on a programme to which, I am thankful to say, I responded.

This was two years ago and now I can get about and kneel much more readily. Though I do get twinges of pain, I haven't had a really bad day with that terrible pain all arthritis sufferers know for over six months. As an added bonus, the colitis is under control, and so is the high blood pressure. I haven't taken a tablet for high blood pressure for over twelve months: my doctor says that the treatment from Mr Rowland is keeping that under control.

Mr V. M. has written a well-documented letter which needs little futher explanation, other than to re-emphasise the importance of sticking to the system as strictly as possible and reaping the rich rewards of good health by doing so.

It is almost six months since I visited the Naturopathic Clinic to consult Mr Rowland about osteo-arthritis which had started to disable me seriously. My feet, legs and hips were painful, the pain extending down my legs and up to my left shoulder and arm. I was unable to sleep and had become almost immobile. The pain was such that I was unable to pick up a cup of tea with my left hand. For four months prior to my consultation with Mr Rowland I had received tablets from my doctor, but as my condition continued to deteriorate I discontinued the tablets.

Mr Rowland prescribed dietary changes, fasting one day a week, herbal medicine, vitamin and mineral therapy and massaging with Rowlo Oil.

AFTER ONE MONTH OF TREATMENT the pain was less intense so that I was able to sleep, and there was a noticeable improvement in my foot joints.

AFTER TWO MONTHS the range of movement in my left arm was considerably better and the pain in my left arm was not so severe. There is now no pain at all in the foot joints. The only areas of pain which remain are the knees, lower back, and hip joints.

AFTER THREE MONTHS I had the full range of movement back in my left arm and shoulder, with only slight pain on waking in the morning. I still have some pain in my back and hip joints but this is considerably less than when I started the treatment.

AFTER FOUR MONTHS there was only slight pain in my back and hip, and shoulder areas.

AFTER ALMOST SIX MONTHS improvement continues. I can walk at almost my old speed, and at sixty-two years of age can move faster than many half my age. The occasional pain I have is only slight.

If you have rheumatoid arthritis then read the following

letter often as it will give you the heart to tackle the condition. Even by keeping to the programme which follows you will find it a battle to overcome the condition; I cannot offer a miracle, merely the means to fight which in itself often results in restored health. Mrs D. was taking a large quantity of tablets and vitamins: this often comes as a surprise to people not previously acquainted with this sort of holistic treatment. There are many reasons for the large quantities of herbal tablets often required and one is that, because the fibres of the plant are left in the tablet, any one tablet contains very little of the active ingredient. Fibres are left in so that, as the tablet disintegrates in the stomach, a wide surface area is created from which the body can extract its requirements. This system means that there will be few or no side effects from what may be a very potent herb: it is this principle on which most of my herbal tablets are formulated.

The other point to look for when reading this letter is the length of time it took for the detoxification to work before any real progress was made and how the vitality was at a low ebb for some considerable time. Gradually, however, the rewards started to come, vitality was restored and the healing process gathered momentum.

Mrs D.'s letter starts with a description of the years of pain from rheumatoid arthritis and the drug therapy with its misery of side-effects and addiction. At the point when her doctors wanted to use yet another drug to help wean her off steroids she turned, at the age of 31 years, to herbal medicine. Her struggle was uphill as she first had to overcome her dependence on Prednisolone. She continues:

With the herbal method certain items were excluded from my diet: white flour, hard fats, white sugar, caffeine and salt. Tablets and medicine were prescribed, special baths were recommended, and I slowly reduced the dose of Prednisolone. After four months I ceased to take Prednisolone at all. I had to suffer all the pains of withdrawal, especially in my back, neck and shoulders, and stiffness in my joints was not confined to mornings, but occurred sometimes during the day as well, being very much in evidence by early evening. This stage lasted for over three months. I needed analgesics during this period and I was very weak, the slightest exertion leaving me shaky and breathless. My tablets were changed, the pain and stiffness eased, and I felt much better. I was able to begin full-time work.

The tablets and medicine were again changed after about six months but did not suit me, and after a while the treatment was changed yet again. In another four months my health was slowly improving, my progress becoming steady. My strength increased and I was at a stage where I could sleep peacefully at night, with only a little stiffness in the mornings, this being wonderful when I think of the time when I had to be helped out of bed. I had greater freedom of movement – once I could not bend down, had difficulty rising from a sitting position and climbing stairs, and even experienced pain in my jaws when eating.

Now four years later my good condition is being maintained and the crippling disease is kept well in control. I am hopeful for the future once more. The people around me seem to have forgotten my illness, although they only knew me after my treatment had started to work: if only they could have seen me in earlier years they would realise that I am indeed living proof that herbal medicine really works.

There is a world of difference in the two types of treatment that I have received – the conventional way with drugs, that I have personally found useless in the long term; and the naturopathic way without harmful side effects and which rebuilds health and strength, revitalising the system.

The interesting point about the success of this next case is that it is the result of a joint effort between myself and the patient's doctor, because she is still on a drug that she finds useful and her doctor prescribes it for her in conjunction with my treatment. My only regret is that her doctor was not standing with me on the first day that she walked from her car leaving her wheelchair behind, a very emotional moment that had my staff crying with joy. The letter which follows is from the client's husband.

Five years ago my wife started to suffer with rheumatoid arthritis; she became very disabled having to use a wheelchair, and she started to stoop. Her arms and legs were very bad. I did not believe in herbalism, but my wife begged me to take her, and so in the end I gave in.

After eighteen months' treatment under Mr Rowland my wife got back the use of her left arm and left leg, and – owing to the skill of Mr Rowland – the arthritis is contained in her left side only, and there is a big improvement in that. Before the start of this treatment my wife could not do anything with her arms, and could not walk a step. Now the stoop is going and she can move her arms; the most amazing thing to me is that she can now walk about 50 yards.

The most interesting aspect of the next letter is how Dr Dong's *Arthritic Cookbook* was being followed with some success but was too severe a regime to stick to for long. This may be the case for some people with my programme and, if in your self-care treatment you feel that you need some encouragement, go without delay to a practitioner who has experience of this type of treatment.

Up to the time I consulted Mr Rowland I had been prescribed pain-killing drugs which relieved the pain of arthritis for only a limited time. I was completely unable to use my hands, drive the car or walk without help.

I then heard of Dr Dong's Arthritic Cookbook and decided to give it a try: after three months most of the pain had gone, along with the swelling, but I didn't feel any better in myself, and I knew that the diet was one I would never be able to keep to.

It was at this point that I decided to pay Mr Rowland a visit: I was very confused about the properties of certain foods and medicines and needed the advice of an experienced practitioner. I had been led to believe that calcium was taboo, as was fruit, but I now know that grapes and pineapple play a big part in helping arthritis, and that calcium pantothenate (Vitamin $B_5$) is essential as it produces necessary hormones and converts carbohydrates into energy.

The salient point of the next letter is contained in just two sentences but is a very important message:

After a few months on Mr Rowland's treatment I found it hard to believe that my worsening symptoms were actually part of the cure, and they would get worse before they got better. However, gradually they abated and I have got better and better, so much so that I now no longer think about my ailments at all and it is difficult to remember how bad they actually were, and how much they got me down.

I leave the last word to Mrs C. who has been attending my clinic for some years now. When she first came to the clinic her condition of osteo-arthritis was quite severe and she was hardly able to walk. Although her progress has been slow it has been steady and now, at the age of 71 years, Mrs C. is living a full and active life, her chief enjoyment being ballroom dancing. The holistic self-care system treats the whole person, restoring vitality and the quest for a new life – which can include ballroom dancing at 71!

I had been under the doctor for six years suffering from osteo-arthritis. I could not walk very much and had a lot of pain. A friend of mine was going to Mr Rowland and took me along: within six weeks I was a little better, and within twelve months I was dancing. I am still dancing at the age of seventy-one.

# 7 The Programme

I have developed this programme of treatment after experience with many hundreds of cases of arthritis of varying degrees of severity. I have found that six distinct stages of progress are achieved and the preparations suitable for each stage are thus different. In the following pages, I outline in brief what you can hope to experience at the six stages, I then give the breakfast and lunch menus to be used throughout the programme, and then deal with the preparations to be used at the six stages of treatment. The ingredients of all the preparations recommended will be found on pp. 77-81.

## THE SIX STAGES OF PROGRESS

1. A feeling that you are more lively and more able to cope with your condition, although the pain has not yet lessened.
2. You are sleeping better and the pain is starting to localise to two or three places.
3. This is a period of very little change and there may even be a slight worsening of the condition, though this will rarely be as bad as before the programme started. This stage may last for several months.
4. A more confident feeling and a slow realisation that you have more mobility.
5. The confidence grows and the pain has almost gone, but there may still be evidence of it in the local areas.
6. Your confidence is fully restored and you start to get

bored with the programme. You can gradually come off the strict guidelines without any ill effects and, because of your re-educated attitude, you will not make many dietary errors in future.

## THE REGULAR MENU

### ON RISING
1 tablespoonful of lemon juice* in a small glassful of water

### BREAKFAST
1 tablespoonful wheatgerm
1 tablespoonful lecithin granules
1 tablespoonful muesli *or* porridge
1 teaspoonful molasses
1 teaspoonful bran
1 teaspoonful honey
Skimmed or raw milk
Wholemeal toast with honey or molasses
Dandelion coffee or decaffeinated coffee

### LUNCH
Salad with plenty of grated root vegetables and sprouting seeds
Fresh fruit (not citrus, except lemon)
Herbal tea
Glass wine if desired

### EVENING MEAL
A good starter is unsweetened pineapple juice.
Rest of the meal is left to your own discretion, but you must follow the general guidelines of the Rowland Remedy Food Guide, as given on pp. 70-76.

* Bottled lemon juice is acceptable, though I prefer the freshly squeezed lemon if available.

It is acceptable to transpose the evening menu with the lunch menu.


## BATHING AND FASTING

There are two particular aspects of the programme that need to be mentioned here.

### SPECIAL BATHS

Twice weekly you should take a special bath, as discussed on p. 24. Add to the bath water ½ lb (250 g) sea salt, ½ lb (250 g) Epsom salts and ½ oz (15 g) powdered culinary ginger. Keep the temperature of the water as high as you can stand throughout the bath by topping up while you are soaking.

When you get out of the bath, lightly dry yourself and apply Rowlo Oil to the whole of the spine and affected areas. Then wrap yourself up well and retire to bed where, hopefully, you will perspire, so aiding the elimination process.

### FASTING

You should fast for 24 hours every seventh day, drinking only grape juice and water.

The way to achieve this is to extend the natural fasting period of sleep and miss first the evening meal on day one, and breakfast and lunch on day two. You will thus create a gap in which eating is allowed on 2 days, but a period of 24 hours without food is nevertheless undergone.

You do not take any preparations during this 24 hour period, but you do have the ones that go with the meals before and after the fast.

Please note in particular that you should keep up the fast all the time you are on the programme, that is, throughout the six stages; you should not have a special bath during the fast period; you may, if you feel at all light-headed during the fast, have a few grapes as well as the grape juice and water.

## STAGE ONE

When you first start taking the preparations as outlined below you may suffer some digestive upset. As my old tutor used to say, 'It is like stirring up a still pond'. If this occurs, go on to the preparations gradually so that you are taking the full amount by the end of the second week. Take the preparations after food and, in the case of the morning and evening meals, take them with the drink made from the tisanes.

I hope that you will have discussed with your doctor your intention to undertake this programme of treatment and that he will co-operate by monitoring your progress for you. It is to be hoped that during this first stage of the programme you can come off any anti-inflammatory or analgesic drugs he may have been prescribing for you.

During this stage you should be getting into the habit of taking the special baths and of undergoing a 24-hour fast every seven days. You will be living with these two aspects of the regime for some time, so some experimentation now with which days of the week best suit your lifestyle will pay dividends over the months.

You should stay on the first stage preparations for at least 42 days before moving on to Stage Two.

## STAGE ONE PREPARATIONS

AFTER BREAKFAST
2 JR Multivitamin and Mineral Formula
1 Vitamin C Plus 500 mg
Parsley Sprinkle
2 Kelp Tablets
Celery Compound Tisane Drink

AFTER LUNCH
2 Pantothenic Acid 500 mg
2 Kelp Tablets

AFTER EVENING MEAL
Parsley Sprinkle
1 Pantothenic Acid 500 mg
2 Kelp Tablets
Celery Compound Tisane Drink

ON RETIRING
1 tablespoonful Cod Liver Oil
2 Meadowsweet and Willow Bark Compound

## STAGE TWO

At this stage you will see that an increased amount of
Pantothenic Acid is stipulated. Also during this stage you
will find that the pain will localise and it is on these local
points that you should use the Rowlo Oil. You will find that
the pain will be different at different times of the day and, if
it becomes difficult to bear, you may take up to 9
Meadowsweet and Willow Bark Compound tablets per day.

This stage will probably go on for 16 to 18 weeks, when
you may well find yourself at something of a standstill. This
signifies the beginning of Stage Three which is a very
important one in the programme.

## STAGE TWO PREPARATIONS

AFTER BREAKFAST
2 JR Multivitamin and Mineral Formula
1 Vitamin C Plus 500 mg
Parsley Sprinkle
2 Kelp Tablets
2 Pantothenic Acid 500 mg
Celery Compound Tisane Drink

After Lunch
2 Kelp Tablets
2 Pantothenic Acid 500 mg

After Evening Meal
Parsley Sprinkle
2 Kelp Tablets
2 Pantothenic Acid 500 mg
Celery Compound Tisane Drink

On Retiring
1 tablespoonful Cod Liver Oil

N.B. You may take up to 9 Meadowsweet and Willow Bark Compound tablets per day if the condition is still painful.


**STAGE THREE**

In Stages One and Two you will have been feeling the benefits of the vitamin, mineral and herbal preparations as well as the improved nutrition from following the food guide. You should be off any toxic medication. This is the point at which the liver will be leading the body to complete detoxification and there may well be withdrawal symptoms and a regression in your condition during this period.

Even if you were not on any prescribed drugs, your body has been asked to do without food substances such as caffeine, sugar and a high salt intake that it may have been used to all your life. These may be the agents that your body is now craving.

It is very important not to weaken in your resolve to attain good health and you should, if anything, become more rigorous in following the Rowland Remedy Food Guide.

During Stage Three, which may go on for weeks or months, the preparations change considerably. We use for the first time Whey tablets and African Devil's Claw, and Jamaican Sarsaparilla and change the tisanes to the formula based on dandelion. You may wish to refer to p. 81 for more information about these substances

## STAGE THREE PREPARATIONS

### AFTER BREAKFAST
2 JR Multivitamin and Mineral Formula
1 Vitamin C Plus 500 mg
1 Whey Tablet 500 mg
1 Pantothenic Acid 500 mg
Parsley Sprinkle
Dandelion Herbal Compound Tisane Drink

### AFTER LUNCH
1 L-Tryptophan 500 mg
1 Whey Tablet 500 mg
1 Pantothenic Acid 500 mg
2 African Devil's Claw and Jamaican Sarsaparilla
   Compound Tablets

### AFTER EVENING MEAL
1 Whey Tablet 500 mg
1 Pantothenic Acid 500 mg
2 African Devil's Claw and Jamaican Sarsaparilla
   Compound Tablets
2 Kelp Tablets
Dandelion Herbal Compound Tisane Drink

### ON RETIRING
1 tablespoonful Cod Liver Oil

N.B. Up to 9 Meadowsweet and Willow Bark Compound Tablets per day may be taken for pain relief.

## STAGE FOUR

You will now have a more confident feeling and your mobility will increase. In particular, your arms may well feel lighter and have more movement.

Together with this greater mobility and increased confidence may come an unexpected pain, and this is the pain of freedom. Your blood circulation will have improved and you will have been through the major part of the detoxification process. There will, however, still be some residual toxic waste in the joints and this will cause pain as you begin to make use of your greater mobility. Do not let this pain concern you; your body will deal with this residual waste matter in good time as long as you persevere with the programme. In the meantime you may find it helpful at this stage to take an additional special bath and to apply the Rowlo Oil more frequently.

## STAGE FOUR PREPARATIONS

AFTER BREAKFAST
2 JR Multivitamin and Mineral Formula
1 Vitamin C Plus 500 mg
1 Whey Tablet 500 mg
Parsley Sprinkle
Celery Compound Tisane Drink

AFTER LUNCH
1 Vitamin E 200 i.u.
1 Pantothenic Acid 500 mg

AFTER EVENING MEAL
1 Whey Tablet 500 mg
1 Pantothenic Acid 500 mg
2 Kelp Tablets
Parsley Sprinkle
Celery Compound Tisane Drink

On Retiring

1 tablespoonful Cod Liver Oil

N.B. Up to 9 Meadowsweet and Willow Bark Tablets per day may be taken if there is still any pain.

## STAGE FIVE

Your confidence will grow markedly during this period as the pain abates and, though there may be some localised pain, your whole general health will be so much improved that you will feel well able to cope.

At this stage you should start to reduce your intake of preparations. I find that people generally find it most tiresome to remember the preparations after the midday meal, so it is probably best to discontinue these first.

## STAGE FIVE PREPARATIONS

After Breakfast

1 JR Multivitamin and Mineral Formula
1 Vitamin C Plus 500 mg
1 Whey Tablet 500 mg
Parsley Sprinkle
Celery Compound Tisane Drink

After Lunch

None

After Evening Meal

2 Pantothenic Acid 500 mg
2 Kelp Tablets
Parsley Sprinkle
Celery Compound Tisane Drink

On Retiring

1 tablespoonful Cod Liver Oil

N.B. If any pain remains Meadowsweet and Willow Bark Tablets may be taken as required, up to a maximum of 9 per day.

## STAGE SIX

At this point you will have achieved a state of relatively good health. You will have become bored with the programme and you can start to come off it. The best way to do this is gradually to relax your lifestyle and not make as many errors as before. In part the programme is educational and, by this stage, you will have found out which of the foods and preparations are most suitable for you.

I recommend that you take the vitamins and minerals and the Celery Compound Tisane Drink at a maintenance level to supplement your diet and any of the other preparations that you feel did you the most good.

## STAGE SIX PREPARATIONS

### After Breakfast
1 JR Multivitamin and Mineral Formula
1 Vitamin C Plus 500 mg
4 Kelp Tablets
Celery Compound Tisane Drink

### After Lunch
None

### After Evening Meal
Any of the preparations that you used in the programme that you felt did you the most good.

### On Retiring
Celery Compound Tisane Drink

# 8 The Rowland Remedy Food Guide

This Food Guide is a quick reference to the foods that you may eat when on the programme. The eight-point plan has been discussed on pp. 60-69, and this has been used to calculate the percentage given to each food. To recapitulate, these factors affecting the suitability of the foods are a high potassium content, a low sodium content, a low sugar content, a high pantothenic acid content, a high fibre content, that the foods should be rich sources of trace elements, and should contain no substances to which you, personally, react badly.

For Stages One to Three you may eat any foods below a 55% rating; for Stage Four any foods below 60%, and for Stages Five and Six, any foods below 70%.

When coming off the diet, the percentage can be increased by 5% per month and each addition to the diet should be studied for adverse reactions. If any present themselves then that food is not for you.

Remember that, although there is no control on the quantity of any food consumed, there are borderline foods which may rate just under your percentage. You must not have too many of these in your overall diet: it should be well-balanced.

## FOOD VALUES

| %   |                       | %   |                         |
|-----|-----------------------|-----|-------------------------|
|     | Almonds               | 50  | Apple juice, bottled    |
| 15  | dried                 | 80  | Apple sauce, sweetened  |
| 75  | roasted, salted       |     | Apricots                |
| 15  | Apple, raw, unpeeled  | 70  | canned                  |

| % | |
|---|---|
| 20 | dried |
| 75 | cooked, sweetened |
| 15 | fresh |
| 75 | nectar, concentrated |
| | Asparagus |
| 75 | canned |
| 40 | frozen spears, cooked |
| 40 | green, cooked |
| 40 | low sodium |
| | Aubergine/Egg plant, |
| 20 | cooked |
| 30 | Avocado pear |
| | |
| 70 | Bacon |
| 95 | Baking powder/soda |
| 15 | Banana |
| 15 | Barley, pearled, light |
| 15 | Bass, sea |
| | Beans |
| 50 | canned |
| 15 | cooked |
| 5 | mung |
| 5 | sprouts |
| | Beef |
| 95 | hamburger |
| 90 | canned roast |
| 85 | corned |
| 85 | dried |
| | lean (grilled, roasted, |
| 75 | braised) |
| 90 | pie, commercial |
| 75 | pie, homemade |
| | stew, canned with |
| 85 | vegetables |
| 75 | stew, homemade |
| | Beet/beetroot |
| 65 | canned, regular pack |
| 50 | cooked |
| 40 | low sodium |
| 60 | Beet greens, cooked |
| | Beverages, alcoholic |
| 80 | bitter beer |
| 30 | lager beer |
| 40 | mild beer |
| 85 | gin |
| 10 | table wine |
| 15 | Blackberries |

| % | |
|---|---|
| 20 | Blueberries |
| 70 | Bouillon cube |
| | Bran with sugar and |
| 75 | malt extract |
| 50 | Bran flakes (40 % bran) |
| 50 | with raisins |
| 10 | Brazil nuts |
| | Breads |
| 20 | cracked wheat |
| 60 | French or Vienna |
| 10 | rye, American |
| 5 | pumpernickel |
| | white, 3-4 % nonfat |
| 80 | milk solids |
| 20 | wholemeal |
| 10 | wholewheat |
| 10 | Broccoli spears |
| 10 | Brussels sprouts |
| | Butter |
| 85 | salted |
| 55 | unsalted |
| 10 | Buttermilk |
| | |
| 20 | Cabbage, cooked |
| 80 | Cakes (home recipe) |
| 85 | angel food |
| 85 | chocolate with icing |
| 45 | fruit, dark |
| 45 | gingerbread |
| 45 | plain without icing |
| 75 | sponge |
| 5 | Carrots |
| 80 | canned, regular pack |
| 45 | cooked |
| 60 | low sodium |
| 5 | Cashew nuts, unsalted |
| | Cauliflower |
| 30 | cooked |
| 5 | fresh |
| 10 | frozen, cooked |
| | Celery |
| 10 | cooked |
| 5 | fresh |
| 80 | Chard, Swiss, cooked |
| | Cheese, half fat |
| 50 | Caerphilly |
| 50 | Cheddar |

| %  |                              |
|----|------------------------------|
| 50 | Cheshire                     |
| 70 | cottage                      |
| 70 | cream                        |
| 50 | Danish blue                  |
| 50 | Edam                         |
| 50 | Gruyère (Swiss)              |
| 20 | Parmesan                     |
| 80 | Cheese, any full fat         |
| 10 | Cherries                     |
| 90 | canned, syrup pack           |
| 50 | frozen                       |
| 10 | Chicken                      |
| 10 | Chicory                      |
|    | Chilli con carne,            |
| 50 | canned with beans            |
|    | Chilli powder with           |
| 50 | seasonings                   |
| 85 | Chocolate, bitter            |
|    | Clams                        |
| 45 | canned                       |
|    | hard, round, meat            |
| 35 | only                         |
| 30 | raw, soft meat only          |
|    | Coconut                      |
| 75 | dried, sweetened             |
| 50 | fresh, shredded              |
|    | Coffee                       |
| 20 | decaffeinated                |
| 85 | instant dry powder           |
|    | Corn                         |
| 90 | rice and wheat flakes        |
| 95 | shredded                     |
| 90 | puffed                       |
|    | Corn, sweet                  |
|    | canned, whole kernel,        |
| 75 | regular pack                 |
| 55 | cooked                       |
| 55 | low sodium pack              |
| 85 | Cornflakes                   |
| 85 | sugar-coated                 |
|    | Cornmeal/polenta or          |
| 70 | maize meal                   |
|    | Cowpeas                      |
| 70 | canned, regular pack         |
| 40 | dry seeds, cooked            |
| 60 | immature, cooked             |
| 35 | Crabmeat, canned             |

| %  |                              |
|----|------------------------------|
|    | Crackers                     |
| 75 | plain                        |
| 75 | soda                         |
| 40 | wholewheat                   |
|    | Cranberry                    |
| 45 | juice                        |
| 45 | sauce                        |
|    | Cream                        |
| 85 | half and half                |
| 90 | light coffee                 |
|    | substitute (cream, skim      |
| 95 | milk, lactose)               |
| 95 | whipping – light             |
| 60 | Cucumbers, not peeled        |
| 75 | Custard, baked               |
|    |                              |
|    | Dandelion                    |
| 10 | coffee                       |
| 10 | greens, cooked               |
| 15 | Dates                        |
| 75 | Doughnuts, cake-type         |
| 15 | Duck, flesh only             |
|    |                              |
|    | Eggs                         |
| 60 | white                        |
|    | whole (no more than 3        |
| 60 | per week)                    |
| 60 | yolk                         |
| 45 | Endive, curly                |
|    |                              |
| 10 | Fats, vegetable              |
|    | Figs                         |
| 20 | canned                       |
| 20 | dried, uncooked              |
| 15 | fresh                        |
| 20 | Flounder                     |
|    | Fruit cocktail,              |
| 20 | fresh                        |
|    |                              |
|    | Gelatine                     |
| 70 | dry                          |
| 75 | sweetened, ready to eat      |
| 10 | Goose, flesh only            |
|    | Grapefruit                   |
| 85 | canned, sweetened            |
| 75 | fresh                        |
| 75 | juice                        |

| %   |                                            | %   |                                         |
| --- | ------------------------------------------ | --- | --------------------------------------- |
| 20  | Grapes                                     |     | Milk                                    |
| 20  | juice, bottled                             | 20  | dry, nonfat, instant                    |
|     |                                            | 80  | evaporated, undiluted                   |
|     | Haddock                                    | 10  | goat's                                  |
|     | fried (dipped in egg,                      | 20  | skimmed                                 |
| 60  | milk, breadcrumbs)                         | 80  | whole pasteurised                       |
| 15  | raw                                        | 85  | Milk beverages                          |
|     | Heart, beef                                |     | chocolate flavoured,                    |
| 80  | cooked, braised                            | 80  | with skimmed milk                       |
| 75  | lean                                       |     | malted with whole                       |
| 15  | Herb teas                                  | 80  | milk                                    |
| 20  | Herring                                    | 30  | Mineral waters                          |
|     | Honey (1 teaspoonful daily                 | 10  | Molasses                                |
|     | only at the start of your                  |     | Mushrooms                               |
|     | programme – no reasonable                  | 70  | canned                                  |
|     | limit when you have reached                | 10  | fresh                                   |
| 50  | 70 in your programme)                      |     | Mustard, prepared                       |
|     |                                            | 65  | yellow                                  |
|     | Ice cream, no added salt,                  | 50  | Mustard greens, cooked                  |
| 60  | approximately 12 % fat                     |     |                                         |
|     |                                            | 20  | Nectarine                               |
| 80  | Jams and preserves                         | 50  | Noodles                                 |
| 80  | Jellies                                    |     |                                         |
|     |                                            | 10  | Oatmeal                                 |
|     | Kale cooked, leaves                        | 60  | cooked, salted                          |
| 10  | with stems                                 | 10  | Oil, vegetable                          |
|     |                                            | 10  | Okra, cooked                            |
|     | Lamb, average of lean                      |     | Olives                                  |
| 75  | cuts, cooked                               | 75  | green                                   |
| 85  | Lard                                       | 60  | ripe                                    |
|     | Lemon juice, fresh                         |     | Onion                                   |
| 50  | (1 daily only)                             | 15  | cooked                                  |
| 80  | Lemonade, frozen, diluted                  | 10  | fresh                                   |
| 20  | Lettuce                                    |     | Orange                                  |
| 75  | Lime juice, fresh or canned                | 70  | juice                                   |
| 75  | Limeade, frozen, diluted                   | 70  | peeled                                  |
|     | Liver, cooked, fried                       | 10  | Oyster                                  |
| 65  | beef                                       |     |                                         |
| 65  | calf                                       | 20  | Papaya, raw                             |
| 55  | pork                                       | 20  | Parsley                                 |
| 25  | Lobster, canned or cooked                  | 20  | Parsnips, cooked                        |
|     |                                            |     | Peach                                   |
| 25  | Macaroni                                   | 55  | canned                                  |
| 70  | with cheese, baked                         | 85  | cooked with sugar                       |
|     | Margarine                                  |     | dried, sulphured,                       |
| 75  | salted                                     | 25  | uncooked                                |
| 20  | unsalted                                   | 10  | fresh                                   |

| % | |
|---|---|
| 50 | frozen |
| 85 | nectar |
| 80 | Peanut butter |
| | Peanuts |
| 50 | roasted |
| 80 | salted |
| | Pear |
| 30 | canned |
| 10 | fresh |
| 95 | nectar |
| | Peas |
| 50 | canned, regular pack |
| 30 | dry, split |
| 30 | frozen |
| 10 | green, cooked |
| 20 | low sodium pack |
| 10 | Pecans |
| | Pepper, sweet, green, |
| 10 | raw |
| 10 | Perch, ocean, Atlantic |
| 10 | Persimmon, Japanese |
| 75 | Pickles |
| | Pies, home recipes, |
| | wholewheat flour |
| 75 | apple |
| 75 | cherry |
| 75 | custard |
| 90 | lemon meringue |
| 90 | mince |
| 70 | pumpkin |
| 70 | Piecrust, baked |
| 50 | Pike, walleye |
| | Pineapple |
| 20 | canned, unsweetened |
| 10 | fresh |
| | juice, canned |
| 10 | unsweetened |
| | Pizza, cheese, home |
| 60 | recipe |
| | Plums |
| 10 | canned, purple |
| 10 | fresh |
| 90 | Popcorn, salted |
| | Pork |
| 70 | fresh, lean, roasted |
| 70 | Picnic ham, lean, simmered |
| | Pork, cured |

| % | |
|---|---|
| 80 | canned, spiced or unspiced |
| | ham, light cure, lean, |
| 70 | cooked |
| | Potatoes |
| 10 | baked |
| 10 | boiled, unsalted |
| 90 | French fried |
| 60 | mashed with milk |
| | potato chips, using |
| 75 | vegetable oil |
| 80 | Pretzels |
| | Prunes |
| 20 | cooked without sugar |
| 20 | dried, uncooked |
| 20 | juice |
| 85 | Pudding, home recipe |
| 85 | bread with raisins |
| 85 | chocolate |
| 85 | cornstarch (blancmange) |
| 85 | rennin, using mix |
| 85 | rice with raisins |
| 85 | tapioca cream |
| | Pumpkin, canned, |
| 30 | unsalted |
| | |
| 20 | Radishes |
| 20 | Raisins |
| 70 | Raspberries |
| 75 | Relish (chutney) |
| | Rhubarb, cooked, |
| 90 | unsweetened |
| 20 | Rice |
| | Rice cereals |
| 70 | flakes |
| 50 | puffed, without salt |
| | Rolls |
| 70 | commercial, plain |
| 70 | sweet |
| 50 | wholewheat |
| 30 | Rye flour, light |
| 70 | Rye wafers |
| | |
| | Salad dressings |
| | commercial mayonnaise |
| 75 | type |
| 75 | French |
| 60 | home-cooked |

| % | |
|---|---|
| 65 | mayonnaise |
| 65 | Thousand Island |
| 10 | Salmon, pink |
| 55 | canned |
| | Sardines, Pacific, canned |
| 50 | in tomato sauce |
| 55 | Sauerkraut |
| 75 | Sausage |
| 75 | Bologna |
| 65 | Frankfurters, raw |
| 70 | pork links, cooked |
| 55 | Scallops, bay, steamed |
| 50 | Shrimp, fresh |
| 80 | Sorbet/sherbert, orange |
| | Soup, canned, diluted |
| | with equal part water |
| 50 | bean |
| 70 | bean with pork |
| 75 | beef bouillon |
| 75 | beef noodle |
| 50 | chicken |
| 50 | clam chowder, Manhattan type |
| 50 | cream soup (mushroom) |
| 50 | lentil |
| 50 | minestrone |
| 50 | onion |
| 50 | pea, green |
| 70 | tomato |
| 80 | vegetable with beef broth |
| 20 | Spaghetti |
| 70 | home recipe |
| | in tomato sauce with |
| 70 | cheese |
| | with tender meatballs, |
| 80 | canned |
| | Spinach |
| 50 | canned, regular pack |
| 15 | cooked |
| 10 | fresh |
| 40 | low sodium |
| | Squash |
| 20 | summer, cooked |
| 10 | winter, cooked |
| | Strawberries |
| 75 | fresh |
| 75 | frozen |

| % | |
|---|---|
| | Sugar |
| 85 | brown |
| 85 | granulated |
| | Sweet potatoes |
| 15 | baked |
| 75 | boiled, candied |
| 85 | Syrup, table blend |
| | Tangerines |
| 70 | fresh |
| 75 | juice, canned |
| 10 | Tapioca |
| 75 | Tea |
| 15 | herb |
| | Tomatoes |
| 75 | canned, low sodium |
| 75 | canned, regular pack |
| 70 | fresh |
| | juice, canned, regular |
| 85 | pack |
| | ketchup, regular |
| 85 | pack |
| 80 | Tongue, beef, braised |
| | Tuna, canned in oil, |
| 55 | solids and liquid |
| | Turkey |
| 15 | dark |
| 10 | light |
| | Turnip |
| 20 | cooked, diced |
| 30 | frozen |
| | greens, canned, regular |
| 40 | pack |
| 10 | Vinegar, cider |
| 85 | Waffles, home recipe |
| 10 | Walnuts |
| 20 | Watermelon |
| | Wheat and malted |
| 55 | barley, dry, cooked |
| 30 | Wheat, rolled, cooked |
| 10 | Wheat bran, crude |
| | Wheat cereals |
| 55 | cooked |
| 65 | flakes |
| 10 | puffed, without salt |
| 10 | shredded, plain |

|   | % | | | % | |
|---|---|---|---|---|---|
| | | Wheat flours | | 55 | White sauce |
| | 55 | all-purpose or family cake | | | |
| | 55 | self-raising | | 10 | Yeast, baker's |
| | 10 | wheatgerm | | | Yogurt, made from par- |
| | 10 | wholewheat | | 10 | tially skimmed milk |

# 9 JR Preparations Guide

**Rowlo Oil**

The Rowlo Oil Formula has benefited a great many of my patients. It is a unique blend of exotic, vegetable and aromatic oils that I combine to help both the arthritic joint and the blood circulation in the soft tissue. It should be applied to the affected joints as required and massaged into the spine as well as the local pain areas after the special baths.

The ingredients are as follows:

Arachis oil *Arachis hypogaea*
Cajuput oil *Melaleuca leucodendron*
Juniper berry oil *Juniperus communis*
Clove oil *Eugenia caryophyllus*
Olive oil *Olea europaea*
Avocado oil *Persea americana*
Amber oil *Pinus palustris*
Almond oil *Prunus communis*
Wintergreen oil *Gaultheria procumbens*


**RR 402    Parsley Sprinkle**

The Parsley Formula is a preparation of finely ground herbs.
The ingredients are as follows:

Parsley *Petroselinum crispum*
Bearberry *Arctostaphylos uva-ursi*
Yarrow *Achillea millefolium*
Prickly ash bark *Zanthoxylum clavis herculis*
Burdock *Arctium lappa*

Poplar bark *Populus tremuloides*
Senna *Cassia angustifolia*
Alfalfa (*Medicago*)


**RR 403    Celery Compound Tisane**

Rheumatic root (wild yam) *Dioscorea villosa*
Yarrow *Achillea millefolium*
Celery *Apium graveolens*
Burdock *Arctium lappa*
Chickweed *Stellaria media*
Willow bark (white willow) *Salix alba*
Alfalfa (*Medicago*)

DIRECTIONS FOR USE
1. Place 2 teaspoonsful in a small teapot.
2. Pour on ½ pint (300 ml) boiling water and stir.
3. Leave to stand overnight.
4. Strain. Take 1 cupful after breakfast and evening meal.


**PR 404    Willow Bark and Meadowsweet Tablets**

When the pain is acute, relief is often gained by an increased
intake of willow bark with meadowsweet added.
White willow bark *Salix alba*
Meadowsweet *Filipendula ulmaria*


**RR 405    Kelp Tablets**

Seaweeds were the first living plants on the earth and there
are over 700 recorded species now in existence. There is
good reason to believe that kelp is one of the first crops to
have been used by Man. It was certainly used by the
Chinese, the Greeks and the Romans not only as a food, but
also as a fertiliser and as a medicine. In Ireland, Wales and
Japan, seaweed is a common food today.

I have found kelp to be beneficial in the treatment of both
over- and underactive thyroid glands, which suggests

a complex make-up of nutrients. I have mentioned earlier that our blood mimics, and therefore resembles very closely, the chemical consistency of sea water. Kelp, in absorbing the nutrients of sea water and processing them into a form that humans can use has done a good job for us. You will not be surprised that kelp tablets are included as a supplement in your total health programme. An average analysis of kelp shows that it contains thirteen vitamins, sixty trace elements and twenty essential amino acids. Please note, particularly if you are a vegetarian, that kelp contains Vitamin $B_{12}$, an ingredient that is often deficient in the vegetarian diet.


### RR 406     Pantothenic Acid Tablets

Each tablet contains 500 mg pantothenic acid (Vitamin $B_5$). (See also p. 100).


### RR 407     JR Multivitamin and Mineral Formula

Although you will not be deficient in very many vitamins and minerals at any one time, by taking this formula regularly you will ensure that you lack none of the vital ingredients for making as speedy as possible a recovery. You should take 2 tablets daily with food.

Each tablet will provide:

VITAMINS

| | |
|---|---|
| Vitamin A (retinol) | 500 µg (1450 i.u.) |
| Vitamin $D_3$ (cholecalciferol) | 4 µg ( 160 i.u.) |
| Vitamin E (dl-α tocopheryl acetate) | 10 mg ( 10 i.u.) |
| Vitamin C (ascorbic acid) | 50 mg |
| Vitamin $B_1$ (thiamine HCl) | 20 mg |
| Vitamin $B_2$ (riboflavin) | 20 mg |
| Vitamin $B_6$ (pyridoxine HCl) | 20 mg |

1 µg = 2.907 international units (i.u.)

| Vitamin $B_{12}$ (cyanocobalamin) | 4 mg |
| Nicotinamide | 20 mg |
| Pantothenic acid | 20 mg |
| d-Biotin | 150 µg |
| Folic acid | 200 µg |
| Para-aminobenzoic acid | 10 mg |
| Choline bitartrate | 10 mg |
| Inositol | 5 mg |

## MINERALS

| Calcium (as phosphate) | 126 mg |
| Phosphorus (as phosphate) | 60 mg |
| Potassium (as phosphate) | 20 mg |
| Magnesium (as oxide) | 25 mg |
| Iron (as ferrous fumarate) | 3 mg |
| Copper (as gluconate) | 100 µg |
| Manganese (as gluconate) | 2.2 mg |
| Iodine (as kelp) | 20 µg |
| Zinc (as oxide) | 1 mg |
| Selenium (as Se yeast) | 25 µg |

## OTHER INGREDIENTS

| Lecithin | 20 mg |
| Betaine HCl | 2.2 mg |
| dl-Methionine | 2.2 mg |
| l-Lysine HCl | 1.75 mg |
| cl-Cysteine HCl | 0.25 mg |
| Glutamic acid | 4 mg |
| Bioflavonoids complex | 5 mg |
| Dried yeast | 20 mg |
| Alfalfa | 20 mg |
| Kelp | 25 mg |
| Ginseng | 20 mg |
| Red Clover | 5 mg |
| *Damiana aphrodisiaca* | 3 mg |

## RR 410    Aly Salt

Aly Salt is potassium chloride. It is an alternative to common sodium chloride, common table salt. It should be used on the food after cooking and not in the original food preparation.


## RR 411    Vitamin C Plus

These tablets each contain 500 mg of ascorbic acid with the addition of 50 mg of the bioflavonoid complex.


## RR 412    African Devil's Claw Tablets

The ingredients are sarsaparilla (*Smilax ornata*) and African devil's claw (*Harpogophytum procumbens*).


## RR 414    Dandelion Herbal Compound Tisane

Yellow dock *Rumex crispus*
Burdock *Arctium lappa*
Wood sanicle *Sanicula europaea*
Buchu *Barosma betulina*
Sarsaparilla (Jamaican) *Smilax ornata*
Skullcap *Scutellaria laterifolia*
Dandelion *Taraxacum officinale*

DIRECTIONS FOR USE
1. Place 2 teaspoonsful in a small teapot.
2. Pour on ½ pint (300 ml) boiling water and stir.
3. Leave to stand overnight.
4. Strain. Take 1 cupful after breakfast and evening meal.


## RR 415    Whey Tablets

The Whey Tablet is a whey concentrate and contains calcium orotate.

## Glossary

| | |
|---|---|
| Alterative | Helps cleanse the system of morbid matter. |
| Anti-bilious | Corrects the bile. |
| Anti-inflammatory | Reduces inflammation. |
| Anti-pyretic | Efficacious against fever. |
| Anti-rheumatic | Relieves rheumatic and arthritic conditions. |
| Antiseptic | Destroys micro-organisms, prevents sepsis. |
| Anti-spasmodic | Relieves or prevents spasm. |
| Carminative | Expels wind. |
| Demulcent | Lubricative. |
| Diaphoretic | Stimulates perspiration. |
| Diuretic | Increases the formation and discharge of urine. |
| Emollient | Causing warmth and moisture. |
| Febrifuge | Dispelling fever. |
| Glycoside | Any group of organic compounds found abundantly in plants which hydrolyse into sugar and other organic compounds. |
| Laxative | Mild purgative. |
| Narcotic | Relieves pain, brings on sleep and, in large doses, coma. |
| Nutritive | Nourishing. |
| Purgative | Promotes bowel action. |
| Resin | A semi-solid substance obtained from exudations of plants. |
| Saponins | Glycosides found in plants which cause water to froth. |
| Sedative | Soothing to the nerves. |
| Stomachic | Strengthens stomach and digestive organs. |
| Tannin | Astringent vegetable compounds. |
| Volatile oil | Odiferous oil obtained from plants containing a variety of chemical compounds. |

# Part 3
# Reference Section

# 10 Herbal Compendium

| | |
|---|---|
| Alfalfa | *Medicago* |
| Almond | *Prunus communis* |
| Amber | *Pinus palustris* |
| Arachis | *Arachis hypogaea* |
| Avocado | *Persea americana* |
| Bearberry | *Arctostaphylos uva-ursi* |
| Bogbean | *Menyanthes trifoliata* |
| Buchu | *Barosma betulina* |
| Burdock | *Arctium lappa* |
| Cajuput | *Melaleuca leucodendron* |
| Celery | *Apium graveolens* |
| Chickweed | *Stellaria media* |
| Clove | *Eugenia caryophyllus* |
| Dandelion | *Taraxacum officinale* |
| Juniper | *Juniperus communis* |
| Kelp | *Laminaria* spp. |
| Meadowsweet | *Filipendula ulmaria* |
| Olive | *Olea europaea* |
| Parsley | *Petroselinum crispum* |
| Poplar bark | *Populus tremuloides* |
| Prickly ash bark | *Zanthoxylum clava herculis* |
| Rheumatic root | *Dioscorea villosa* |
| Sarsaparilla | *Smilax ornata* |
| Senna | *Cassia angustifolia* |
| Skullcap | *Scutellaria laterifolia* |
| Willow bark | *Salix alba* |
| Wintergreen | *Gaultheria procumbens* |
| Wood sanicle | *Sanicula europaea* |

Yarrow           *Achillea millefolium*
Yellow dock     *Rumex crispus*

## Alfalfa                      *Medicago*

*Constituents:* Source of vitamins, mineral salts, potassium, phosphorus, iron.
*Action:* Nutrient.

Alfalfa is a rich source of nutrients, particularly potassium, phosphorus, and iron, which are obtained by the roots of the plant which extend deep into the ground, sometimes as much as 40 feet (12 m). It has recently become a popular food supplement for people on fitness programmes and those who are convalescing.

## Almond                 *Prunus communis*

*Constituents:* Fixed oil, consisting mainly of olein and a small proportion of linolein.
*Action:* Nutrient and demulcent.

Most people will be familiar with the almond nut, if not the oil, but we use both at some stage of the programme. The oil is one of the ingredients in Rowlo Oil which is used for the massage after the special baths and the nut will be found in the muesli.

The almond tree is mainly found in warm climates but it has always been popular in gardens in temperate climates.

The nutritive value of the nut has made it popular with naturopaths who frequently recommend that ten almonds be taken daily, chewed well.

## Amber                  *Pinus palustris*

*Constituents:* Properties similar to those of turpentine oil and is obtained by the distillation of certain resins or by distilling resin oil.

Amber oil (*Oleum succini*) is one of the ingredients in Rowlo Oil. It has long had a reputation for its healing properties and is included in many liniments throughout the world.

### Arachis                                   *Arachis hypogaea*
*Constituents:* Fixed oil, proteins, starch.
*Action:* Nutritive, emollient.

The peanut is familiar worldwide both as a nut and as peanut butter. The oil is one of the ingredients in Rowlo Oil and has a beneficial effect on inflamed joints. On its own it is liable to go rancid, but as an ingredient in a blend of oils it lasts well.

### Avocado                                   *Persea americana*
*Constituents:* Edible oil, the fruit has a high protein and potassium content.

Due to a highly successful cultivation and marketing programme, the avocado pear has become commonplace throughout the world and is now included in most recipe books.

I have found the oil to be of great benefit: it has a distinct cooling effect and it was for this reason that I decided some years ago to include it in the Rowlo Oil formula.

### Bearberry                              *Arctostaphylos uva-ursi*
*Constituents:* Tannin, acids, glycosides.
*Action:* Urinary antiseptic, astringent, diuretic, anti-inflammatory.

Virtually all the past and present-day herbal pharmacies would have *uva-ursi* or bearberry leaves in stock. It has certainly been used in the UK since the thirteenth century for conditions associated with inflammation of the urinary organs and its ability to act as an efficient diuretic.

It combines well with other herbs to form effective compounds.

## Bogbean                           *Menyanthes trifoliata*

*Constituents:* Volatile oil, glycosides and bitters.
*Action:* Tonic, bitter, diuretic.

Bogbean is also referred to as buckbean and marsh trefoil. It is almost a specific herb for the treatment of arthritis and almost always appeared as part of the medicine chests in the monasteries, particularly in Germany where the plant has been held in high esteem for centuries.

I have been including this herb in my arthritis formula for some years now with excellent results and I refer to it as my bogbean compound.

## Buchu                              *Barosma betulina*

*Constituents:* Volatile oil and an agent called diosphenol which has antiseptic qualities.
*Action:* Urinary antiseptic, diuretic, diaphoretic, anti-inflammatory.

I have found the beneficial effects of this herb to be tremendous; it has undoubted powers as a urinary antiseptic and I have achieved remarkable results by basing a formula on buchu for such conditions as cystitis, gravel and inflammation of the bladder, as well as arthritis. In fact, I had an enquiry from one of Britain's leading hospitals asking how I had successfully treated a patient of theirs with whom they had had little success. I explained that I was using a herb that was first introduced into medicine in this country in 1821 and was, for over a hundred years, the official treatment for cystitis, urethritis and catarrh of the bladder. With the advent of antibiotics it lost its popularity but not its usefulness; it is still as useful today as it was in 1821.

**Burdock** *Arctium lappa*

*Constituents:* Inulin, bitters, resin, fixed and volatile oils, flavonoids, anti-bacterial substances.

*Action:* Mild diuretic, anti-bacterial, alterative.

Burdock was used by the herbalists in their treatment for gonorrhea before the advent of antibiotics. It has always been regarded as a strong alterative or blood cleanser and is today used in treatments for arthritis, gout, eczema and psoriasis and is often used in conjuction with slippery elm bark in treating anorexia nervosa.

Apart from its contribution to herbal medicine, burdock has two other claims to fame: the first one is the burrs which are the plant's means of disseminating itself, hence the various synonyms by which it is referred to throughout the world such as thorny burr, beggar's buttons or hoppy major. It is also one of the basic ingredients of that popular drink, dandelion and burdock.


**Cajuput** *Melaleuca leucodendron*

*Constituents:* Volatile oil.

*Action:* Anti-spasmodic, diaphoretic, stimulant, antiseptic.

The cajeput tree, which is a native of the East Indies, has produced for us one of the finest volatile oils that are at present available for use in our treatment programme. When applied externally it is a stimulant and mild counter-irritant. When taken internally, it has a highly stimulant action, producing an increased pulse rate and often profuse perspiration. In moderate doses it is used for conditions such as laryngitis, bronchitis and cystitis.


**Celery** *Apium graveolens*

*Constituents:* Two oils, volatile and fixed.

*Action:* Anti-rheumatic, sedative, diuretic, urinary antiseptic, carminative.

I hold celery in high esteem and have used the seeds, prepared in various forms, as part of a treatment programme for many conditions, not just arthritis. I have found the celery aids the nervous system and helps promote a healthy sleep which is beneficial whatever your condition. Although we use the seeds in a concentrated form, please also include celery in your diet as often as possible.

## Chickweed                                    *Stellaria media*
*Constituents:* Saponins.
*Action:* Anti-rheumatic, alterative, antiseptic, demulcent.

Chickweed spread around the world at about the same rate that the world became Westernised, and so will be familiar to most people reading this book. It has been used in herbal medicine for internal preparations and for Chickweed Ointment which is particularly useful for conditions of the skin.

## Clove                                      *Eugenia caryophyllus*
*Constituents:* Volatile oil.
*Action:* Stimulant, carminative, aromatic.

The clove's medicinal properties are chiefly held in the volatile oil, the taste and smell of which will almost certainly be familiar to you. Externally it is best combined with other oils as it is in Rowlo Oil.

Internally it has long been used as an aid to the digestive process particularly in relieving flatulence. It may be applied directly on the gums to stop them bleeding. Recently it has started once again to be used as a natural preservative.

## Dandelion                                   *Taraxacum officinale*
*Constituents:* Bitters, taraxacerin, glycosides, potassium.

*Action:* Anti-rheumatic, diuretic, anti-inflammatory, mild laxative.

The dandelion is a familiar plant to us all and a particularly useful one, both for its edible and medicinal properties. It gets its name from a corruption of the French name 'dent de lion' because the leaves have a jagged appearance that resembles the teeth of lions.

The leaves are used in salads and they have a slightly bitter taste when young. They are often used boiled as a substitute for spring cabbage or spinach. The plant is popular as a partner in that famous drink dandelion and burdock. The roots are roasted to form dandelion coffee – a very pleasant drink which I recommend as an excellent substitute for tea or ordinary coffee. The absence of caffeine is a bonus to anyone on a detoxification programme.

The history of dandelion as a medicinal plant goes back hundreds if not thousands of years. There are many early references in India to dandelions being most suitable for liver complaints. This is probably because the root contains a bitter substance called taraxacerin which is active against diseases of the liver.

It is also beneficial to the kidney and urinary systems and is a general stimulant to the system.

Apart from its uses in compounds for arthritis, herbalists would use it for such conditions as cholecystitis, gall stones and jaundice.


**Juniper** *Juniperus communis*

*Constituents:* Volatile oil, bitters, organic acids.

*Action:* Anti-rheumatic, diuretic, anti-inflammatory antiseptic, stomachic.

Juniper berries have been used in medicine, both herbal and allopathic, since early Greek and Roman times. The oil is chiefly used both internally for indigestion, flatulence, and diseases of the kidney and bladder, and externally, combined with other oils, as a mild stimulant for arthritic and skin conditions.

## Kelp
*Laminaria* spp.

*Constituents:* A wide range of minerals and trace elements, the most important being iodine.

*Action:* Protects against infection, regulates and activates metabolism.

See pp. 78-79 for details of this substance.

## Meadowsweet
*Filipendula (Spiraea) ulmaria*

*Constituents:* Essential oil with salicylic acid compounds.

*Action:* Anti-rheumatic, aromatic, astringent, diuretic, antacid, antiseptic.

Meadowsweet is often referred to as 'queen of the meadow' and is one of the best known wild flowers, probably due to the overall fragrance of the plant. It is unusual because the scent of the leaves is different from that of the flowers and gives much pleasure to our sense of smell.

It has been a favourite ingredient of herb beers since medieval times and there were few monasteries that did not include meadowsweet in their medicine chest, where they would use it in compounds for disorders of the stomach and bowels, and for arthritis, probably due to its salicylic content.

## Olive
*Olea europaea*

*Constituents:* Oil, resin.

*Action:* Antiseptic, astringent, febrifuge, demulcent, mild laxative.

My chief interest in olive is the use of the oil in Rowlo Oil and for taking internally, combined with lemon juice, as a tonic to the liver.

You will undoubtedly be familiar with olive oil, but perhaps not aware of the process which is used for extraction. The first pressing of the fruit is achieved by crushing the olives in rough bags which are immersed in water. The oil which floats on the water is skimmed off and this oil has a slight green tint and is referred to as 'virgin' or 'first pressing'. This is available in most good shops and is the one that we want for our programme.

To obtain the second pressing of the oil, the cake is moistened and allowed to ferment: this is not the quality for us.

**Parsley**                                    *Petroselinum crispum*

*Constituents:* Essential oils, apiol, glycosides, Vitamin C.
*Action:* Aperient, diuretic, carminative.

This herb needs little in the way of description as it is widely used in cookery throughout the world. It originally became popular as a culinary herb because it is one of the richest sources of Vitamin C.

This may contribute to its diuretic action, i.e. helping the body to reduce its excess water.

It combines well with other herbs to make effective herbal compounds, particularly where there may be any congestion of the kidneys.

**Poplar Bark**                                *Populus tremuloides*

*Constituents:* Salicin, populin.
*Action:* Anti-rheumatic, antiseptic, febrifuge, anti-inflammatory.

This was undoubtedly one of the essential herbs to be included in the medicine chest of the monasteries. It was often combined with meadowsweet for fevers, sciatica and pains of the hip.

**Prickly Ash Bark**                    *Zanthoxylum clava herculis*

*Constituents:* Volatile oil, alkaloids.

*Action:* Anti-rheumatic, stimulant, carminative, alterative, tonic.

The prickly ash bark is highly regarded in the USA for use in countering arthritis, skin conditions and impurities of the blood. The early settlers used the powdered bark on varicose ulcers and for cleaning old wounds. It was also made into a tonic for the system which was used in debilitating conditions of the stomach and digestive organs, such as colic and cramp. There is much interest amongst the herbal community in prickly ash due to its stimulant action which helps in circulatory conditions, such as intermittent claudication and Raynaud's syndrome.


**Rheumatic Root**                    *Dioscorea villosa*

*Constituents:* Steroidal, glycosides, saponin.

*Action:* Anti-rheumatic, anti-inflammatory, mild diaphoretic.

There are over 150 varieties of *Dioscorea* and herbalists gave this one the name of rheumatic root to distinguish it from the rest. Its other name is wild yam.

It is not only an important anti-rheumatic herb, being almost a specific for arthritis, but is also particularly useful for any internal inflammation, such as cholecystitis or diverticulitis, and is also helpful in circulatory conditions such as intermittent claudication.

Its more recent claim to fame is the fact that we obtain from it the agent diosgenin which is the precursor for the manufacture of steroids and the contraceptive pill.


**Sarsaparilla (Jamaican)**                    *Smilax ornata*

*Constituents:* Saponins, glycosides.

*Action:* Anti-rheumatic, antiseptic, alterative.

Sarsaparilla is famous as a drink which is often sold alongside dandelion and burdock, each having their own distinct flavour. It is one of the strongest alteratives that we have and its powers for cleansing the blood and giving a clear skin are renowned.

It was first introduced into the UK in the sixteenth century for the treatment of syphilis and other venereal diseases, and in all probability will soon be required again as antibiotics are now starting to be non-effective in this area of disease. More recently it has been used for other chronic conditions, such as arthritis, where it is still popular to this day in herbal medicine.

## Senna                                    *Cassia angustifolia*
*Constituents:* Anthraquinone and derivatives.
*Action:* Purgative.

Senna is undoubtedly the best known of any of the herbs mentioned for this programme, its purgative action being well known for hundreds of laxative preparations.

In our programme we use the fruit of the senna, the pods, which are not quite as severe in their actions as the leaves.

Senna originated in Egypt and has been cultivated in the UK since 1640.

## Skullcap                                 *Scutellaria laterifolia*
*Constituents:* Flavonoid glycosides, volatile oil, tannin, bitters.
*Action:* Sedative, anti-spasmodic.

Before stronger synthetic sedatives came onto the market, skullcap was considered to be almost a specific for the convulsive twitchings of St Vitus' Dance.

It still has a tremendous following amongst insomniacs as a pleasant way of inducing sleep without any of the unpleasant side effects of synthetic drugs.

The anti-spasmodic effect of skullcap has ensured its place in the folklore of Europe and the USA for its ability to cure hiccups.

## Willow Bark                                   *Salix alba*
*Constituents:* Tannin, salicin.
*Action:* Anti-rheumatic, anti-inflammatory, antiseptic, analgesic, anti-pyretic.

Willow bark is an excellent source of salicin which is closely related to aspirin (which is in fact acetylsalicylic acid). It is probably for this reason, and the tannin content, that this herb has gained its high reputation.

In the treatment programmes, this herb is combined with meadowsweet.

## Wintergreen                          *Gaultheria procumbens*
*Constituents:* Volatile oil containing methyl salicylate.
*Action:* Stimulant, astringent, aromatic.

We are particularly interested in wintergreen for its volatile oil content which is one of the ingredients in Rowlo Oil. It has a particularly beneficial effect when combined with other oils and applied externally to the affected areas. It is also a useful oil for sportsmen to apply to the muscles to avoid mid-game cramp and maintain supple muscles.

## Wood Sanicle                            *Sanicula europaea*
*Constituents:* Tannin, bitters.
*Action:* Astringent, alterative, anti-inflammatory.

The origin of the name sanicle is the Latin word 'sano', 'heal or cure'.

In the Middle Ages, it gained a high reputation for treating conditions of the blood, being said to cleanse the body of morbid material, leaving the blood healthier and in better condition. This is just right for the arthritis programme where detoxification is the main theme.

It is often combined with other herbs rather than used on its own.

### Yarrow                                    *Achillea millefolium*
*Constituents:* Volatile oil, glyco-alkaloid, tannin.
*Action:* Diuretic, diaphoretic, anti-pyretic, astringent, hypotensive.

Yarrow has a wonderful reputation throughout the world of herbal medicine for its ability to combine well with other herbs. On its own it is almost a specific for disorders of the circulatory system and arthritic conditions.

It has long been a favourite herb of mine, particularly when combined with rutin.

### Yellow Dock                                    *Rumex crispus*
*Constituents:* Glycosides, tannin.
*Action:* Laxative, alterative, anti-rheumatic.

Yellow dock contains the same glycoside (hydroxy-anthraquinone) as senna which accounts for its laxative powers, but it also contains other agents which make the overall effect of this herb not as searching as senna. It is a useful blood purifying agent and makes an excellent member of a compound to treat arthritis and skin diseases.

# 11 Vitamins

Here we look at the vitamins with which you are likely to come into contact when on a a treatment programme. For each of the vitamins current to date, I have outlined the relevant data, function, natural sources and deficiency manifestations. I have also made a personal comment as to the attention you need to pay to ensure you have an adequate supply of each vitamin.

Vitamins are a group of substances essential to life which are found in foodstuffs. They are potent organic compounds, although they are found only in very small concentrations. For a substance to be classified as a vitamin, it must firstly perform specific functions in the cells and body tissues; secondly, the body must be unable to synthesise sufficient for its needs; and thirdly, its absence would result in a deficiency disease.

An important point which you should understand is that vitamins found in nature work synergistically, that is, they work together creating a greater force than the sum of their parts. This co-operation is found in many areas, but one very noteable synergistic action is that of the B complex vitamins. Thus, although it is acceptable to take a single Vitamin B factor as a supplement it is necessary to ensure that your intake of the whole B complex is adequate.

**Vitamin A**

Fat soluble.
Measured in micrograms (μg).
Retinol is Vitamin A.

Carotene precursor is converted to Vitamin A at a ratio of 6:1.

Works in conjuction with Vitamin D.

*Functions:* maintains healthy epithelial cells, mucous membranes, skin and bone.

*Natural sources:* liver, egg yolk, dairy produce, vegetables, apricots, cod liver oil.

*Deficiency manifestations:* dry mucous membranes, loss of taste and smell, rough or dry skin, glare or night blindness.

*Note:* an important vitamin, especially for the health of the eye. It is as well to pay particular attention to your intake of this vitamin if you are a smoker, or watch a lot of television or if you spend a lot of time under fluorescent light.

The fact that this vitamin is fat-soluble means that it can build up in the liver and, if too much is taken, Vitamin A toxicity can result.

You obtain Vitamin A direct from foods as retinol, or from the substance called carotene which the body converts to Vitamin A.

## Vitamin $B_1$     Thiamine

Water-soluble, thus excess is excreted by body and regular intake required.

Measured in milligrams (mg).

Tissues of the heart, liver, brain and kidneys have the highest concentrations in the body.

*Functions:* essential for growth. Aids digestion and the conversion of carbohydrates into energy. Improves confidence. Aids the muscles and nerves, particularly the heart muscles, in functioning correctly.

*Natural sources:* wheat germ, nuts, beans, whole grains, pulses, dairy foods,

*Deficiency manifestations:* nervous disorders, irritability, brain fag, easy exhaustion, poor digestion, depressed state.

*Note:* you may recall reading in your history books about the disease beri beri, caused by a severe deficiency of Vitamin B. Until the discovery of the cause of the condition by Dr Edward Vedder in the Philippines in 1910, this disease was responsible for many deaths. Dr Vedder cured babies dying of beri beri by giving them rice bran.

The subsequent discovery of the Vitamin $B_1$ was made by Dr R.R. Williams and from this discovery stemmed the ability to synthesise the vitamin. This largely eradicated the disease. It should be re-emphasised, however, how important bran or fibre can be in our diets.

If you are a smoker or a drinker then you will almost certainly need plenty of thiamine. People who have a high sugar intake may also be at risk of a deficiency.

## Vitamin $B_2$     Riboflavin

Water-soluble and, though the body storage is slightly better than thiamine, a daily intake is still indicated.
Measured in milligrams (mg).
Stable to heat, acid and oxidation.
Sensitive to alkali.
Should be stored in the dark as it is destroyed by light when in solution.

*Functions:* essential to a number of chemical reactions in the body for the release of energy within the cell, thus growth, and for healthy skin, gums and eyes.

*Natural sources:* wheatgerm, liver, soya beans, eggs, vegetables, milk, cheese, fish.

*Deficiency manifestations:* nervousness, irritability, dry hair, dry skin, mouth ulcers, ocular problems such as frontal headaches, eye strain, itching and sensitivity to light.

*Note:* riboflavin functions as part of a group of enzymes called flavoproteins which are vital to the metabolism of carbohydrates, fats and proteins. It also has an important role to play in the health of the eye.

### Vitamin B$_3$      Niacin

Water soluble.
Measured in milligrams (mg).
Stable in dry state, even in alkali.
Comes in two forms: nicotinic acid and nicotinamide.

*Functions:* involved in the synthesis of proteins and fats, therefore helpful to healthy skin, the gastro-intestinal tract and nervous system. Helps reduce cholesterol deposits.

*Natural sources:* liver, lean meats, whole grains, fish, eggs, nuts, dates, prunes.

*Deficiency manifestations:* pellagra, a disease which affects the skin, digestive system and nervous system

*Note:* niacin, nicotinic acid and nicotinamide have nothing at all to do with nicotine as found in tobacco.

The body's requirements are uncertain, though it seems to obtain its supplies by converting the amino acid tryptophan into niacin. This process requires the presence of pyridoxine (Vitamin B$_6$), an example of the need to ensure the presence of all the B Vitamins.

### Vitamin B$_5$      Pantothenic Acid

Water soluble.
Measured in milligrams (mg).

*Functions:* part of a co-enzyme which plays a role in the metabolism of carbohydrates, fats and proteins, allowing the release of energy. Aids in the synthesis of amino acids, the body's basic building blocks, fatty acids, sterols, and steroid hormones. Essential to the formation of porphyrin, the pigment portion of the haemoglobin molecule.

*Natural sources:* liver, kidney, heart, wholewheat bread, brown rice, salmon, eggs, nuts, broccoli.

*Deficiency manifestations:* hair loss, grey hair, dry skin, digestive disorders.

*Note:* the word 'pantothenic' means widespread, which gives you some idea of the importance put on this vitamin by nature.

Pantothenic acid plays a vital role in the programme of treatment because of its function in aiding the synthesis of amino acids, the sterols and the body's own steroid hormones which are essential for the body to be able to heal itself.

A high pantothenic acid content is one of the factors in the eight-point Rowland Remedy Food Guide.

## Vitamin $B_6$     Pyridoxine
Water soluble and regular supply needed due to poor retention by the body.
Measured in milligrams (mg).
Stable to light and oxidation.
Considerable losses occur in refining, or in heating food above boiling point.

*Functions:* essential for healthy muscle, skin and nerves. Enables the body to use protein more efficiently, also to convert tryptophan to niacin.

*Natural sources:* glandular meats, lamb, legumes, potatoes, oats, wheatgerm, bananas. Some may be found in vegetables such as cabbage and carrot.

*Deficiency manifestations:* muscle cramps, anaemia, irritability, depression. In cases of severe shortage, the onset of convulsions and formation of kidney stones may present.

*Note:* I have prescribed pyridoxine over a long period for problems associated with the menopause, particularly the depressive state. The most successful dose seems to be 300 mg daily.

A regular dose of 100 mg daily, throughout the cycle, is sufficient for other disorders, such as pre-menstrual syndrome, and I recommend between 50 mg and 100 mg regularly if oral contraceptives are being used.

### Vitamin B$_{12}$  Cyanocobalamin (Cobalamin)

Water soluble.

Measured in micrograms (µg).

Stable during cooking.

*Functions:* A co-enzyme in many of the chemical reactions in the cell, and has a major role to play in the formation of red blood cells in the bone marrow. The nerve cells and the skin also require it for proper function.

*Natural sources:* liver, eggs, sea food.

*Deficiency manifestations:* anaemia, nervous debility, poor concentration, memory loss and lack of energy.

*Note:* the body's requirements of this vitamin are very small and it should not be taken in excess. It works in conjunction with folic acid. As with all the B vitamins it is better when taken synergistically, that is, in balance with the others in the group.

The main cause of the deficiency diseases seems to be malabsorption in the small intestine, and great attention should be paid to improving the health of the intestines, for example by taking a good supply of yogurt.

If you are using the contraceptive pill, if you smoke, or if you are a vegetarian you may well need extra Vitamin B$_{12}$ in your diet. Strict vegetarians will need to rely on comfrey or kelp, or take this vitamin in supplement form.

### Vitamin B Group  Folic Acid

Water soluble.

Measured in micrograms (µg).

*Functions:* essential for the formation of blood, the growth and division of cells and a healthy digestive process.

*Natural sources:* green vegetables, liver, milk, yeast, wheatgerm, soya flour.

*Deficiency manifestations:* diarrhoea, anaemia, depression, glossitis, stomach distension.

*Note:* folic acid works in conjuction with Vitamin E so it is important to take them together. Together they help the assimilation of pantothenic acid which is highly important in the treatment of arthritis. Coeliacs, users of the contraceptive pill, and pregnant women should pay particular attention to their intake of folic acid.


**Vitamin B Group    PABA (Para-aminobenzoic Acid)**
Water soluble.
Measured in milligrams (mg).
Form of folic acid.
Very closely related to the B complex, but as it may be synthesised by bacteria in the intestine it is, strictly speaking, not a vitamin.

*Functions:* helps maintain healthy skin and hair. Essential in the formation of folic acid.

*Natural sources:* brewer's yeast, whole grains.

*Deficiency manifestations:* psoriasis, eczema.

*Note:* this is one of the best sunscreens we can use, so it is an important ingredient in any good ointments for protection against sunburn.


**Vitamin B Group    Biotin**
Water soluble.
Measured in micrograms (μg).
The intestinal bacteria are able to produce biotin, thus it is not strictly a vitamin.

*Functions:* essential for the metabolism of proteins, the proper function of the digestive process and in achieving healthy hair.

*Natural sources:* liver, mushrooms, whole grain rice, brewer's yeast, soya beans, bananas, egg yolks, green vegetables.

*Deficiency manifestations:* anorexia, depression, debility, muscular pain, anaemia, a possible increase in cholesterol.

*Note:* raw egg whites seem to the major enemy of biotin, although food processing and alcohol are close behind.

You will have no deficiency of this substance if you are following the Rowland Remedy Food Guide.


**Vitamin B Group      Choline**
Water soluble.
The body is able to manufacture its own choline from the amino acid methionine as long as sufficient $B_{12}$ and folic acid are present.

*Functions:* when combined with inositol it helps in the dispersal of fats and fat soluble vitamins throughout the body.

*Natural sources:* liver, lecithin, brewer's yeast, fish, soya beans, wheatgerm, vegetables.

*Deficiency manifestations:* loss of memory, poor concentration, senile dementia, poor co-ordination.

*Note:* extra choline should be added to your diet in the form of lecithin if you consume alcohol or are on the contraceptive pill.


**Vitamin B Group      Inositol**
Water soluble.
Measured in milligrams (mg).
*Functions:* combined with choline it helps in the dispersal of fats throughout the body.

*Natural sources:* liver, lecithin, brewer's yeast, fish, soya beans, whole grains, wheatgerm, vegetables.

*Deficiency manifestations:* poor concentration, poor memory co-ordination, brain fag, senile dementia.

*Note:* inositol is sensitive to water, alcohol, caffeine and the contraceptive pill.

Always try to think of inositol with choline, as they have a combined role to play in nature.


### Vitamin $B_{13}$    Calcium Orotate

Water soluble.

Measured in milligrams (mg).

*Functions:* aids cell regeneration, glandular function, proper function of the liver and pancreas. It is linked with metabolising folic acid and Vitamin $B_{12}$.

*Natural sources:* milk whey, root vegetables.

*Deficiency manifestations:* gout, excessive uric acid deposits.

*Note:* as milk whey is often difficult to obtain, the best source is as a supplement of calcium orotate tablets.

I would recommend Vitamin $B_{13}$ for high blood pressure, as a sports supplement, and for alcoholics who are drying out. It is unquestionably helpful in liver conditions such as hepatitis and cirrhosis.


### Vitamin $B_{15}$    Pangamic Acid

Water soluble.

Measured in milligrams (mg).

An anti-oxidant similar in action to Vitamin E.

*Functions:* helps create healthy blood and tissues, mainly by improving the transportation of oygen to the cell and improving muscle tissue.

*Natural sources:* rice bran, maize, oatflakes, wheatgerm.

*Deficiency manifestations:* brain fag, debility, night cramps, lack of muscle tone.

*Note:* there is some doubt about whether this substance is essential to life and therefore whether it should have vitamin status, although it is beyond doubt that it is helpful to the body. It certainly helps the blood circulation by improving the supply of oxygen to the cell and, because of this, athletes from all over the world have been taking supplements of pangamic acid for many years now.

It can help with all conditions that require improved circulation, such as diabetes, hypertension, angina, thrombosis, asthma and arthritis. If taken in supplement form, it is important to establish that it is derived from natural sources and not synthetic in origin. If you are on the treatment programme, your intake is guaranteed as this substance is found in foods recommended in the menu, such as bran, oats and wheatgerm.


## Vitamin C    Ascorbic Acid

Water soluble, thus not stored well by the body.
Measured in milligrams (mg).

*Functions:* helps to form the intercellular substance collagen necessary for cellular oxidation and reduction. Improves the body's defence mechanisms.

*Natural sources:* citrus fruits, blackcurrants, strawberries, green vegetables, potatoes, cauliflower.

*Deficiency manifestations:* scurvy, skin diseases, bleeding gums, sensitive mouth and gums, capillary fragility.

*Note:* although Vitamin C is probably the best commonly known vitamin there is still much research being done to determine whether high doses might be useful in the prevention and cure of diseases hitherto not associated with the vitamin, such as cancer.

## Vitamin D       Calciferols

Fat soluble.

Calciferol measured im micrograms (μg).

Vitamin D measured in international units (i.u).

1 μg calciferol = 40 i.u.

Vitamin D is really a complex and has at least 10 associates. Two of the most important ones are $D_2$ or ergocalciferol, and $D_3$ or cholecalciferol. $D_2$ is formed when ultra-violet light is passed over the pro-vitamin, or precursor, ergasterol, which is found in the lower forms of plant life, such as yeasts and fungi, $D_3$ is formed when ultra-violet light is passed over the pro-vitamin cholestrol, which is found in the skin and other tissues. Vitamin D is often referred to as the 'sun vitamin' because of the need for ultra-violet light in its formations.

*Functions:* essential for the absorption of calcium and phosphorus, and subseqeunt utilisation for bone growth by regulating the calcium levels in the blood.

*Natural sources:* fish, dairy products, cod liver oil.

*Deficiency manifestations:* rickets, soft bones, poor teeth, skeletal deformities.

*Note:* a very important vitamin for any programme dealing with a degenerative disease. Vitamin D works closely with Vitamin A. I favour cod liver oil and sunlight as the best source of this vitamin.

## Vitamin E

Fat soluble.

Measured in international units (i.u.) or milligrams (mg).

d-α tocopherol 1 mg = 1.49 i.u.

d-α tocopheryl acetate 1 mg = 1.36 i.u.

d-α tocopheryl acid succinate 1 mg = 1.21 i.u.

dl-α tocopherol 1 mg = 1.1 i.u.

dl-α tocopheryl acetate 1 mg = 1 i.u.

dl-α tocopheryl acid succinate 1 mg = 0.89 i.u.

The naturally-occurring tocopherols have the prefix d.
The synthetic tocopherols have the prefix dl.
Tocopherol is the alcoholic form.
Tocopheryl is the ester form.

*Functions:* improves blood circulation, prevents and dissolves blood clots. Acts as an antioxidant in the body, protecting the polyunsaturated fats in the cell walls from peroxidation, thus essential to all life processes.

*Natural sources:* wheatgerm, green vegetables, vegetable oils, legumes, peanuts, wheatgerm oil.

*Deficiency manifestations:* poor circulation and fatigue are two signs, but a deficiency will manifest itself in many different diseases associated with degeneration of the body.

*Note:* Vitamin E has long been known as the anti-sterility vitamin. Care should be taken not to take too much if you are inclined to high blood pressure. If you are on a treatment programme you will be receiving enough.


**Vitamin K**

Fat soluble.

Synthesised by bacterial activity in the intestine.

*Functions:* essential to the formation of the factors associated with the clotting of blood.

*Natural sources:* liver, green vegetables, dairy produce, vegetable oils, soya beans.

*Deficiency manifestations:* slow clotting of blood and lack of prothrombin.

*Note:* this vitamin is found in abundance and you can be sure of receiving your body requirements from a mixed diet.

# 12 Minerals and Trace Elements

**Calcium     Symbol Ca     Atomic Weight 40**

There is a greater weight of calcium in the body than of any other mineral and most of it is in the bones and teeth. It is essential for their strong growth and maintenance. It is equally necessary for sound sleep and strong nerves, an undersupply often resulting in muscle spasms and cramp. Adequate Vitamin A must be available for calcium to be assimilated. Calcium has a balanced relationship with magnesium and phosphorus (see below for details of these minerals).

*Sources:* milk and milk products, cheeses, sardines, nuts, beans, green vegetables. Dolomite tablets (calcium and magnesium in a correct balance) and bonemeal tablets taken with Vitamin A provide good suplements.


**Chlorine     Symbol Cl     Atomic Weight 35.5**

As Chlorides

Associated with sodium and potassium it is required to keep the body fluid's near-neutrality. Chlorine as hydrochloric acid in the stomach aids the digestion of food.

*Sources:* an excess, in the form of sodium chloride, is more likely than a deficiency (see also sodium below).

As Chlorinated Water Supply

Chlorine is used to destroy bacteria. If the excess chlorine is not removed by boiling, it can reduce Vitamin E levels and useful bacteria in the stomach. This can be remedied by taking supplements of Vitamin E and taking plenty of yogurt.

## Chromium    Symbol Cr    Atomic Weight 52
Chromium is essential to the body's utilisation of carbohydrates. There is evidence to support the theory that diabetes may be caused by a deficiency of this element, perhaps by reducing the tissue response to insulin.

*Sources:* meat, shellfish, chicken, whole grains, seeds, brewer's yeast. Multi-mineral supplements contain chromium.

## Cobalt    Symbol Co    Atomic Weight 59
Cobalt is contained in Vitamin $B_{12}$ which is the term used to describe a number of cobalamin compounds. These have proved useful in the treatment of pernicious anaemia.

*Sources:* cobalt as Vitamin $B_{12}$ is found only in food of animal origin and deficiences, though very rare, may occur in strict vegetarians. Supplements are available and Vitamin $B_{12}$ is normally included in a B complex supplement.

## Copper    Symbol Cu    Atomic Weight 64
Copper is a constituent of all human tissues, with the highest concentrations in the brain, liver, kidneys, heart and pancreas. It is essential for the metabolism of iron in the synthesis of haemoglobin and for the utilisation of Vitamin C and of the amino acid tyrosine. It maintains energy by aiding effective iron absorption.

Most foods contain traces of this element, so deficiency is rare.

*Sources:* dried beans, peas, prunes, wholewheat, calf and beef liver, sea food.

## Fluorine    Symbol F    Atomic Weight 19

This element belongs to the same group as chlorine, bromine and idodine. It is widely distributed in human tissues, with the highest concentrations found in the teeth and bones. It improves the resistance of the tooth enamel to acids, thus reducing dental caries.

Fluorides are readily absorbed but only slowly excreted in the urine, and so can cause cumulative toxicity. An excess can mottle the teeth.

*Sources:* sea food. In many areas, there is controlled addition of fluoride to the drinking water (1 p.p.m.). Before taking additional fluoride you should check with your water authority to find out what the level in your area is.

## Iodine    Symbol I    Atomic Weight 127

This element belongs to the same group as chlorine, bromine and fluorine. It is concentrated in the body in the thyroid gland and influences its activity, thus controlling the metabolism. It provides energy and promotes growth, healthy hair, skin and nails.

Iodides are rapidly absorbed and rapidly excreted in the urine but the thyroid is capable of absorbing enough for its requirements very quickly.

Solutions of iodine are use externally as disinfectants.

*Sources:* iodine is widely distributed in nature, as metallic iodides, in very low concentrations.

## Iron    Symbol Fe    Atomic Weight 56

As an element essential to the production of haemoglobin, it is vital to life. Most of the body's iron is found in the blood (as haemoglobin), but it is also needed for muscle pigment (myoglobin) and certain enzymes. The liver, spleen and bone marrow contain iron.

The assimilation of iron requires an adequate presence of the elements copper, cobalt and manganese, and also Vitamin C.

Anaemia is normally associated with iron deficiency.

*Sources:* liver, kidneys, red meat, egg, oatmeal, nuts, beans. Iron supplements should be the organic acid salts, e.g. gluconate, fumarate or palmitate for best assimilation. Iron salts of inorganic acids, e.g. iron sulphate, are less well assimilated and can be harmful to Vitamin E. The iron must be in the reduced ferrous state; in the oxidised ferric state the iron cannot be absorbed.

## Magnesium    Symbol Mg    Atomic Weight 24

Magnesium is essential for the stability of the neuro-muscular system, but in high concentrations it can act as a depressant. It is necessary also for healthy muscle since the muscle enzymes cannot metabolise sugar without it.

It is needed for the assimilation of calcium and phosphorus. A balance between calcium and magnesium exists in a ratio of approximately 2:1 in the body, and an excess of either should be avoided. Magnesium deficiency may cause the deposition of calcium in the soft tissues.

Vitamin $B_6$ is essential for normal levels of magnesium in the blood and tissues, and magnesium activates many enzymes containing Vitamin $B_6$. Neither nutrient can function in the absence or deficiency of the other.

*Sources:* lemons, grapefruit, nuts, apples, green vegetables. If supplements are to be taken, they are best in the form of salts of organic acids rather than magnesium sulphate, because magnesium is absorbed only with difficulty in the gastro-intestinal tract – to the extent, in fact, that it acts as a laxative.

## Manganese    Symbol Mn    Atomic Weight 55

This is an essential trace element, related to vanadium and chromium, found widely in human tissue, particularly in blood, liver, kidney, pancreas and hair. It is necessary for the utilisation of important B vitamins and the function of the central nervous system. It affects the function of the pancreas and a lack of it can lower the glucose tolerance level. It is an essential co-factor in the function of many enzymes. A high calcium and phosphorus intake requires extra manganese.

*Sources:* nuts, green leaf vegetables, whole grain cereals, oats, rye, peas, beans, dried fruits, raspberries and tea. Manganese is available in synthetic form in mineral supplements.

## Molybdenum    Symbol Mo    Atomic Weight 96

An essential trace element, related to chromium, and present in soils and sea water. It aids in carbohydrate and fat metabolism and there are indications that the presence of molybdenum improves the utilisation of iron.

*Sources:* vegetables, wheatgerm, fish and other marine-based foods including kelp and sea salt. Synthetic supplements are not recommended because of the possibility of toxicity.

## Phosphorus    Symbol P    Atomic Weight 31

Phosphorus is necessary to the life process in every body

cell and for the growth and maintenance of good teeth and bones. The intake must be balanced with the intake of calcium otherwise the excess is excreted as calcium-phosphorus salts, depleting the body's reserve of calcium.

Too much iron and magnesium in food can reduce the assimilation of phosphorus by precipitation of insoluble phosphates in the intestine.

Phosphorus aids in the metabolism of fats and starches and in the assimilation of niacin.

*Sources:* fish, poultry, meat liver, brewer's yeast, lecithin, eggs, nuts. These should be taken in conjunction with calcium-rich foods.

### Potassium      Symbol K      Atomic Weight 39

The elements potassium and sodium regulate the body's water balance. With the element chlorine, as chloride ion, they maintain the body fluids' near-neutrality. An excess of either potassium or sodium is undesirable, leading to an upset in the body fluid balance.

Potassium activates many enzymes essential for good nerve and muscle function and is necessary also for converting carbohydrates into energy or into body starch (glycogen) for storage.

*Sources:* vegetables, fruits, whole grains, nuts and meats. Potassium is fairly widely distributed in foods and the requirements should be adequately covered by a well-balanced diet. Remember, though, that a high intake of salt can result in a high potassium loss, as can prolonged periods of mental and physical stress.

### Selenium      Symbol Se      Atomic Weight 79

This element belongs to the same group as sulphur. It is essential to life and widely distributed in tissues, blood and the main organs.

Selenium is synergistic with Vitamin E in preventing ageing and the hardening of tissues. Liver necrosis and muscular dystrophy may be associated with a selenium deficiency, though this rarely occurs on a good diet.

*Sources:* tuna, herring, brewer's yeast, wheatgerm, bran, onions, cabbage, tomatoes.


### Sodium    Symbol Na    Atomic Weight 23

See potassium, above, for importance of sodium-potassium balance. Instances of high blood pressure are often associated with an excess of sodium.

*Sources:* Sodium is so widely distributed in foods, particularly in convenience foods, that the daily intake is more than likely to be in excess of requirements. In abnormal conditions, however, for example when prolonged exposure to heat or long periods of physical exercise result in excessive perspiration, too much sodium may be lost from the body. Additional salt must be taken under these circumstances to prevent heat exhaustion.


### Sulphur    Symbol S    Atomic Weight 32

Sulphur is ingested mainly in the form of sulphur-containing amino acids. e.g. methionine, cysteine and cystine. Methionine is very important as a basis for the synthesis of many essential compounds in the body. The sulphur-containing amino acids are essential for the production of tissue proteins, e.g. keratin, which keeps the nails, skin and hair healthy. They are also involved in the detoxification of aromatic compounds such as benzene.

Sulphur is used as a bactericide in ointments.

*Sources:* beef, beans, eggs, fish, cabbage

**Vanadium     Symbol V     Atomic Weight 51**

An essential trace element present in soils and sea water. Its essential role is thought to be the control of formation of cholesterol deposits in the arteries.

*Sources:* fish and other marine-based foods, including kelp and sea salt. Although excess vanadium is rapidly excreted from the body, synthetic supplements are not recommended because of the possibility of toxicity.

**Zinc     Symbol Zn     Atomic Weight 65**

Whole blood contains a significant quantity of zinc, mainly in the red cells. An adequate supply is necessary for the action of at least twenty enzymes, one of them, in the retina of the eye, being responsible for Vitamin A metabolism (one type of night blindness appears to be due to a zinc deficiency).

High concentrations of zinc are found in the pancreas: it is released at the same time as insulin and appears to prolong its action.

Zinc deficiency can result from a diet high in phosphorus which impairs zinc absorption. Growth and sexual development can be affected, resistance to infection can be lowered, healing impaired and a skin condition similar to psoriasis can result.

*Sources:* shellfish, lamb, pork, brewer's yeast, pumpkin seeds, eggs. Supplements are available and zinc salts such as gluconate, lactate and citrate are preferred to salts of inorganic acids such as sulphate.

# 13 Foodstuffs

### Bran

Bran is the hard, outer skin of the wheat grain. Although it contains significant quantities of protein, carbohydrate, calcium and iron they have little nutritional value as bran is indigestible in the human alimentary tract. It is, however, this very property which gives it a value as a good source of dietary fibre which, by speeding the passage of waste materials through the bowel, helps to minimise constipation.

Bran is frequently included in weight-reducing diets because of its water retention property which gives a feeling of a full stomach.

### Honey

You will have observed that I recommend honey as opposed to sugar as the sweetener for breakfast. It has many properties that we should make full use of on a health programme.

When the forager bee moves from blossom to blossom, it collects the nectar and pollen and transports them back to the hive, where the mixture is transferred (from bee to bee) and, in the process, the moisture content is reduced until it is concentrated into what we know as honey.

Because it is a simple sugar it does not need digesting and is suitable for infant feeding. It has been used for this purpose for over 2000 years. Its healing, antiseptic and germicidal properties are also renowned.

117

A major Russian scientist attributes the long life of the Bulgarian peasants to their reliance on honey as a food and it would seem appropriate, on this assumption alone, that we include it in our health programme, but we know that, apart from any special properties, it also contains essential vitamins and minerals such as potassium, calcium, magnesium, iron, chloride, sodium, silicon, silica, manganese, sulphur, phosphorus and copper. All of this makes it not only a food fit for 'Kings and Gods', as the ancient philosophers used to refer to it, but also suitable to be included in our fitness programme.

### Milk

Milk, it should be remembered, is a food for babies and infants and should not be taken in excess by adults.

The milk that is consumed on this programme should be very limited in quantity and be skimmed, goat's, or raw, in that order of preference. Raw milk is untreated milk from herds which have been accredited free from TB and brucellosis.

As we are striving in the programme to reduce the overall intake of fat, then it must follow that skimmed milk is the most suitable for the diet.

One further point worth mentioning is that milk is not easily digestible on its own due to the formation of curds in the stomach. It is best used mixed with other foods, preferably starch in some form, e.g. muesli, porridge, rice or bread pudding.

### Molasses

Molasses is considered by many to be a wonder food: it is certainly one of nature's richest sources of vegetable iron which is vital to maintaining good health and energy.

Molasses is the residue left behind when sugar is being

refined and it is rich not only in iron but also in vitamins and minerals, in particular potassium which is one of the main reasons for including it in the regular breakfast in the programme.

Many of my patients have been unable to take the molasses in the breakfast mixutre and have found it better to take on toast or as a drink. Either way is acceptable.

### Muesli

In the early twentieth century, the Swiss dietitian, Dr Bircher-Benner, thought that one should start the day with a highly nutritious breakfast that was easy to prepare and had the health-giving properties of fibre, natural nutrients and the properties of milk that are known to help the digestive tract stay healthy. He combined oats, millet and wheat with hazel nuts, almonds and fresh apple and added a little lemon juice with honey and milk to taste. This provided all the nutrients that the body would need to start the day.

Today there are many brands of muesli available in the shops, all of them based on the original concept of Dr Bircher-Benner. You will see from the programme that muesli is used as the base for the Rowland Remedy breakfast. However, I do appreciate that some people react badly to muesli and, in these circumstances, I recommend porridge as a base. See below for details of oats.

### Oatmeal

Oats are the edible grain from the cereal grass, *Avena sativa*, which is used by herbalists for its muscle- and body-building properties and as a nerve tonic. Oatmeal is one of the most nutritious of the cereals, but surprisingly is not widely used. It has a well balanced protein, fat and

119

carbohydrate content, giving it a high energy value. It is also a useful source of Vitamin $B_1$ and iron.

Its energy value is best obtained as oatcakes. As porridge, it is easily digested but its energy value per serving is significantly reduced by the dilution with water.


### Salads

All the usual vegetable ingredients of a salad, for example lettuce, celery, onions, peppers, tomatoes and cucumber, have a low energy value. The main nutritional value of salads lies in their vitamin A, potassium and iron content and they should always be made up with fresh ingredients.


### Sprouting Seeds

Seeds contain the concentrated energy to enable a plant to survive during its early growth. The sprouting seeds contain vitamins and nutrients in a live, growing state, as opposed to vegetables and fruits that have been harvested for an unknown period, are no longer fresh and have deteriorated to some degree.

Sprouting seeds can be cultivated at home and suitable seeds and instructions can be purchased at health food stores.

One of my favourite sprouting seeds is mung bean sprouts. These are exceptionally high in nutrients, particularly potassium. The nutrients are in an easily absorbable form during the period that the beans are sprouting and they are thus a highly desirable food.


### Vegetables, Root and Tuber

The reason I recommend the use of root vegetables in salads is for their energy and nutritive values, the roots being the plants' storehouse of sugars and starches. There are also many health properties ascribed to roots. Beetroot, for instance, is reputed to be an excellent food for the red blood corpuscles and is the reason why it is the basis for a naturophatic approach to treating various forms of cancer, with the juice from 1.5 kg of the fresh roots being consumed daily by patients who are on special diets for this condition.

Carrots are another favourite root of mine, the juice being of great value in many conditions, due to the concentrations of the precursor β-carotene and other nutrients. They can be of help not only to people who have arthritis but also to those who suffer from conditions such as obesity, high blood pressure, colitis and poor eyesight, among others. The maximum benefits can be obtained from the carrot by extracting the juice or shredding the raw flesh as part of a salad.

Another well known root is horseradish (*Armoracia rusticana*), a highly concentrated food which stimulates the appetite by aiding the secretion of gastric juices. It has the reputation of being a solvent for any excess of mucus in the system, so it is especially useful to include in your diet when you have a cold or catarrh, and perhaps asthma. Do not eat too much, however, as it can be irritating to the kidneys and bladder.

The Jerusalem artichoke is the tuber of the *Helianthus tuberosus* plant and is a very worthwhile food, particularly for diabetics who have to watch the overall amount of carbohydrate in their food.

Onions are of special interest to us on this health programme as they are not only high in potassium but also have undisputed antiseptic properties and are helpful in draining the cavities of mucus, so helping in the detoxification sections of our treatment.

Parsnips (*Pastinaca sativa*) have long been recommended for sufferers of arthritis and should be used in your diet as often as possible. They should be cooked only briefly.

Sweet potatoes are the edible tubers of *Batatas batatas*, They are a rich source of vitamins and minerals, being particularly rich in phosphorus and potassium. They are easily digested and have beneficial effects on people with delicate digestive processes, stomach ulcers and inflamed conditions such as colitis. They can be prepared for eating in much the same way as the white potato.

The white potato is the edible tuber of *Solanum tuberosum* and is so well known that it need not be dealt with in any detail, except to say that I have often recommended the juice of the white potato to be drunk three times daily on an empty stomach for stomach ulcers. This was a recommendation of a friend of mine, Dr A. Vogel, made some years ago when he was paying me a visit and I have passed on the advice to the great benefit of a lot of people.

### Water

In view of the fact that our body weight is made up of 70% fluid, I feel that we should pay some attention to the type of water that we drink.

Water, being nature's solvent, is essential to the proper working of the body. It is necessary to have an adequate (regular) intake of water for the kidneys to work efficiently, i.e. 1-1.5 litres as liquid and approximately 1 litre as food. The digestive process relies on water to work efficiently and so does the skin for its many functions. Due to the regular loss of fluid by the body (about 2 litres per day) it is important to replace this amount on a daily basis.

In most western countries, the tap water is safe due to the bactericides that are added, but I nevertheless recommend a home water-filter system which may be purchased at very low cost. It will give you good clear water for drinking or for making herbal teas, or for ice cubes or for cooking. It removes the chalk, scum, taint and the dissolved gases that we do not want and leaves behind the minerals and trace elements that are so important to good health.

The alternative is bottled mineral waters that are now becoming popular all over the world: you will be drinking water with healthy properties, at the same time eliminating the need to drink from the local supply.

The EEC rules for classifying a mineral water require that nothing can be added or taken away; the only exceptions are the separation of the unstable elements, such as iron and sulphur compounds. This may be achieved by filtering or decanting methods with the strict proviso that the basic composition of the water is not altered. They also require that the water be from an underground source that is bacteriologically pure and of constant composition.

All water contains nitrate, which in excess can be harmful to babies as it can change to nitrite in the body and interfere with the transfer of oxygen in the bloodstream. To obviate this, the EEC permits a maximum level of nitrate of 50 mg per litre for all waters whether tap or bottled.

The sodium content is also controlled at a maximum of 175 mg per litre, as it is generally accepted that high salt levels are undesirable.

You will have gathered that I am keen on having a home filter system and using bottled mineral waters whenever possible. Here are details of some mineral waters available on the market.

**Apollinaris** (Bad Neuenahr, West Germany) Named after St Apollinaris, it has a naturally sparkling, slightly alkaline, taste with a high mineral content.
**Ashbourne** (Derbyshire, Peak District, England) Due to the fact that the UK has no naturally sparkling springs, this water is available both in its still form and also artificially carbonated.
**Badoit** (St Galmier, France) A lightly sparkling water from deep in the Alps with a high calcium and magnesium content. Refer to pp. 109 and 112 for more information on these minerals.

**Contrex** (France) This is a still water, high in minerals, which also has natural diuretic properties.

**Evian** (Mont Blanc, France) A still water with a low mineral content.

**Highland Spring** (Perthshire, Scotland) Like Ashbourne water, this is available in its natural still form or artificially carbonated.

**Malvern** (Malvern Hills, England) Available in both still and carbonated forms.

**Perrier** (Vergeze, South of France) A favourite all over the world. It has a natural sparkle created by past volcanic activity which has dissolved the gases in Perrier which includes traces of xenon, crypton, argon, neon and helium.

**San Pellegrina** (Italy) This has a high mineral content and has been artificially carbonated to make an ideal dining accompaniment.

**Spa** (Belgium) A popular low-mineral water that is available in its naturally sparkling form or in a still form for regular use.

**Vichy Celestins** (France) Has a high sodium bicarbonate content which has made it a popular guest at a rich meal. I have many patients who order this water by the crate because they are so impressed by the aid it has given their digestive system.

**Vichy St Yorre** (France) Has a slight sparkle and is gaining popularity as a top quality table water.

**Vittel** (France) A still water which has an overall low mineral content but is high in calcium and magnesium and therefore has all the benefits of these minerals (see pp. 109 and 112).

**Volvic** (Auvergne Mountains, France) A still water, low in minerals.


## Wheatgerm

Wheatgerm is the part of the grain that is needed for the wheat to germinate. It is the life force of the grain and a rich source of concentrated nutrients. It contains Vitamins A, E and the B group, also copper, magnesium, manganese, calcium and phosphorus as well as other trace elements. It is thus included in the breakfast programme.

It is usually available in two forms. The first is the completely unprocessed raw form, which is certainly the best source of the nutrients but which is more susceptible to rancidity. This form should be refrigerated for storage and used up quickly.

Probably the safer form is stabilised, or toasted, wheatgerm which keeps for a much longer period and has a pleasanter taste. It also should be refrigerated once opened, preferably in an airtight container.

### Wholemeal, Wholewheat, Wheatmeal Flour

There is often a degree of confusion about the different types of brown flour available. In the main there are two types of brown flour: a) wholewheat, wholemeal or 100% wholemeal and b) wheatmeal.

You can immediately see where the confusion arises, especially when the prefix 'stoneground' appears on many packets of flour on the shelves today. So let us take a closer look. Wholewheat, wholemeal and 100% wholemeal are all whole grain flour using 100% of the wheat grain, including the bran and the wheatgerm. The word to be looking for is 'whole'.

Wheatmeal, on the other hand, has either 15% or 19% of the bran (depending on which type of wheat is used) removed to give a smoother flour. It is therefore better for you than white flour but not so nutritious as wholewheat flour.

Many of the flours on sale are described as being stone-ground. This means that the flour was made by rotating two stones at slow speeds. This process has many advantages over the newer steel roller mills in that the stones maintain the grain at a lower temperature and therefore preserve the heat-sensitive nutrients, such as Vitamin E, for the consumer's benefit.

# Index

Numbers in *italics* refer to illustrations